Anonymizing Health Data

Khaled El Emam and Luk Arbuckle

Beijing • Cambridge • Farnham • Köln • Sebastopol • Tokyo

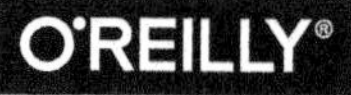

Anonymizing Health Data

by Khaled El Emam and Luk Arbuckle

Printed in the United States of America.

Published by O'Reilly Media, Inc., 1005 Gravenstein Highway North, Sebastopol, CA 95472.

O'Reilly books may be purchased for educational, business, or sales promotional use. Online editions are also available for most titles (*http://my.safaribooksonline.com*). For more information, contact our corporate/institutional sales department: 800-998-9938 or *corporate@oreilly.com*.

Editors: Andy Oram and Allyson MacDonald
Production Editor: Nicole Shelby
Copyeditor: Charles Roumeliotis
Proofreader: Rachel Head
Indexer: WordCo Indexing Services
Cover Designer: Randy Comer
Interior Designer: David Futato
Illustrator: Rebecca Demarest

December 2013: First Edition

Revision History for the First Edition:

2013-12-10: First release

2014-08-13: Second release

See *http://oreilly.com/catalog/errata.csp?isbn=9781449363079* for release details.

ISBN: 978-1-449-36307-9

[LSI]

Table of Contents

Preface

Although there is plenty of research into the areas of anonymization (masking and de-identification), there isn't much in the way of practical guides. As we tackled one anonymization project after another, we got to thinking that more of this information should be shared with the broader public. Not an academic treatise, but something readable that was both approachable and applicable. What better publisher, we thought, than O'Reilly, known for their fun technical books on how to get things done? Thus the idea of an anonymization book of case studies and methods was born. (After we convinced O'Reilly to come along for the ride, the next step was to convince our respective wives and kids to put up with us for the duration of this endeavor.)

Audience

Everyone working with health data, and anyone interested in privacy in general, could benefit from reading at least the first couple of chapters of this book. Hopefully by that point the reader will be caught in our net, like a school of Atlantic herring, and be interested in reading the entire volume! We've identified four stakeholders who are likely to be specifically interested in this work:

- Executive management looking to create new revenue streams from data assets, but with concerns about releasing identifiable information and potentially running afoul of the law
- IT professionals who are hesitant to implement data anonymization solutions due to integration and usability concerns
- Data managers and analysts that are unsure about their current methods of anonymizing data and whether they're compliant with regulations and best practices
- Privacy and compliance professionals who need to implement defensible and efficient anonymization practices that are pursuant with the relevant regulations in their jurisdiction

Conventions Used in this Book

The following typographical conventions are used in this book:

Italic
: Used for emphasis, new terms, and URLs.

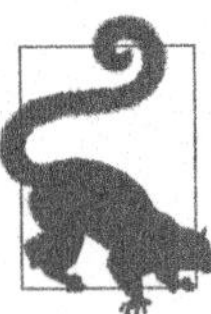

This element signifies a tip, suggestion, or a general note.

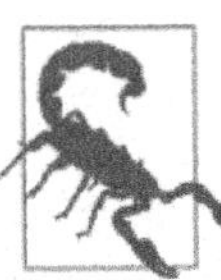

This element indicates a trap or pitfall to watch out for, typically something that isn't immediately obvious.

Safari® Books Online

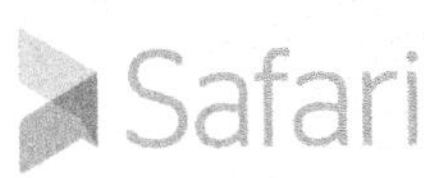

Safari Books Online is an on-demand digital library that delivers expert content in both book and video form from the world's leading authors in technology and business.

Technology professionals, software developers, web designers, and business and creative professionals use Safari Books Online as their primary resource for research, problem solving, learning, and certification training.

Safari Books Online offers a range of product mixes and pricing programs for organizations, government agencies, and individuals. Subscribers have access to thousands of books, training videos, and prepublication manuscripts in one fully searchable database from publishers like O'Reilly Media, Prentice Hall Professional, Addison-Wesley Professional, Microsoft Press, Sams, Que, Peachpit Press, Focal Press, Cisco Press, John Wiley & Sons, Syngress, Morgan Kaufmann, IBM Redbooks, Packt, Adobe Press, FT Press, Apress, Manning, New Riders, McGraw-Hill, Jones & Bartlett, Course Technology, and dozens more. For more information about Safari Books Online, please visit us online.

How to Contact Us

Please address comments and questions concerning this book to the publisher:

O'Reilly Media, Inc.
1005 Gravenstein Highway North
Sebastopol, CA 95472

800-998-9938 (in the United States or Canada)
707-829-0515 (international or local)
707-829-0104 (fax)

We have a web page for this book, where we list errata, examples, and any additional information. You can access this page at *http://oreil.ly/anonymizing-health-data*.

To comment or ask technical questions about this book, send email to *bookquestions@oreilly.com*.

For more information about our books, courses, conferences, and news, see our website at *http://www.oreilly.com*.

Find us on Facebook: *http://facebook.com/oreilly*

Follow us on Twitter: *http://twitter.com/oreillymedia*

Watch us on YouTube: *http://www.youtube.com/oreillymedia*

Content Updates

August 2014

Chapter 1, Introduction
: This chapter includes a new section on automating the anonymization of data sets, and describes how this will increase the number of anonymization professionals by making the methods accessible to a broader and less specialized audience.

Chapter 2, A Risk-Based De-Identification Methodology
: We have provided new guidance on selecting direct and indirect identifiers, including a decision tree to simplify the process.

Chapter 13, De-Identification and Data Quality: A Clinical Data Warehouse
: Here, we consider the before and after effects of anonymizing a clinical data warehouse—specifically, two study protocols that are of interest to researchers and a closer look at date shifting.

Acknowledgements

Everything accomplished in this book, and in our anonymization work in general, would not have been possible without the great teams we work with at the Electronic Health Information Lab at the CHEO Research Institute, and Privacy Analytics, Inc. As the saying goes, surround yourself with great people and great things will come of it. A few specific contributors to this book should get a high five: Andrew Baker, an expert in algorithms, for his help with covering designs and geoproxy risk; Abdulaziz Dahir, a stats co-op, who helped us with some of the geospatial analysis; Aleksander Essex, a wizard in cyber security and applied cryptography, for helping develop the secure linking protocol; Ben Eze and his team of merry developers that put code to work; Youssef Kadri, an expert in natural language processing, for helping us with text anonymization; and Ann Waldo, a legal expert on privacy, information security, and health care issues.

Of course, a book of case studies wouldn't be possible without data sets to work with. So we need to thank the many people we have worked with to anonymize the data sets discussed in this book: BORN Ontario (Ann Sprague and her team), the Healthcare Cost and Utilization Project, Heritage Provider Network (Jonathan Gluck) and Kaggle (Jeremy Howard and team, who helped organize the Heritage Health Prize), the Clinical Center of Excellence at Mount Sinai (Lori Stevenson and her team, in particular Cornelia Dellenbaugh, sadly deceased and sorely missed), Informatics for Integrating Biology and the Bedside (i2b2), the State of Louisiana (Lucas Tramontozzi, Amy Legendre, and everyone else that helped) and organizers of the Cajun Code Fest, the American Society of Clinical Oncology (Joshua Mann and Andrej Kolacevski), IMS Brogan (Neil Corner and his team) for their help with the data quality analysis, and the Public Health Agency of Canada (Tom Wong and his team) as well as Jay Mercer at the Bruyere Hospital and family clinic for working with us on the chlamidya protocol.

Finally, thanks to the poor souls who slogged through our original work, catching typos and helping to clarify a lot of the text and ideas: Andy Oram, technical editor extraordinaire; Jean-Louis Tambay, an expert statistician with a great eye for detail; Bradley Malin, a leading researcher in health information privacy; David Paton, an expert methodologist in clinical standards for health information; and Darren Lacey, an expert in information security. It's no exaggeration to say that we had great people review this book! We consider ourselves fortunate to have received their valuable feedback.

CHAPTER 1

Introduction

Anonymization, sometimes also called *de-identification*, is a critical piece of the healthcare puzzle: it permits the sharing of data for secondary purposes. The objective of this book is to walk you through practical methods to produce anonymized data sets in a variety of contexts. This isn't, however, a book of equations—you can find those in the references we provide. We hope to have a conversation, of sorts, to help you understand some of the problems with anonymization and their solutions.

Because the techniques used to achieve anonymization can't be separated from their context—the exact data you're working with, the people you're sharing it with, and the goals of analysis—this is partly a book of case studies. We include many examples to illustrate the anonymization methods we describe. Each case study was selected to highlight a specific technique, or to explain how to deal with a certain type of data set. They're based on our experiences anonymizing hundreds of data sets, and they're intended to provide you with a broad coverage of the area.

We make no attempt to review all methods that have been invented or proposed in the literature. We focus on methods that have been used extensively in practice, where we have evidence that they work well and have become accepted as reasonable things to do. We also focus on methods that we've used because, quite frankly, we know them well. And we try to have a bit of fun at the same time, with plays on words and funny names, just to lighten the mood (à la O'Reilly).

To Anonymize or Not to Anonymize

We take it for granted that the sharing of health data for the purposes of data analysis and research can have many benefits. The question is how to do so in a way that protects individual privacy, but still ensures that the data is of sufficient quality that the analytics are useful and meaningful. Here we mean proper anonymization that is defensible: anonymization that meets current standards and can therefore be presented to legal authorities as evidence that you have taken your responsibility toward patients seriously.

Anonymization is relevant when health data is used for secondary purposes. Secondary purposes are generally understood to be purposes that are not related to providing patient care. Therefore, things such as research, public health, certification or accreditation, and marketing would be considered secondary purposes.

Consent, or Anonymization?

Most privacy laws around the world are consent-based—if patients give their consent or authorization, the data can then be used for the purposes they authorize. If the data is anonymized, however, then no consent is required. In general, anonymized data is no longer considered personal health information and it falls outside of privacy laws. Note that we use the term "personal health information" to describe the broad universe of identifiable health information across the world, regardless of regulatory regime.

It might seem obvious to just get consent to begin with. But when patients go to a hospital or a clinic for medical care, asking them for a broad consent for all possible future secondary uses of their personal data when they register would generally be viewed as coercive, because it wouldn't really be informed consent. These concerns could be mitigated by having a coordinator discuss this with each patient and answer their questions, allowing patients to take consent forms home and think about it, or informing the community through advertisements in the media. But this could be an expensive exercise to do properly, and would still raise ethical concerns if the permissions sought were very open-ended.

Furthermore, in some jurisdictions (like the EU) personal information must be "collected for specified, explicit and legitimate purposes and not further processed in a way incompatible with those purposes," according to the Data Protection Directive 95/46/EC. This has been interpreted to mean that the purpose of the data processing must be specified somewhat precisely, and that further processing must not be incompatible with the purposes for which personal data were originally collected.[1] This raises a question about the legitimacy of broad consent.

When you consider large existing databases, if you want to get consent after the fact, you run into other practical problems. It could be the cost of contacting hundreds of thousands, or even millions, of individuals. Or trying to reach them years after their health care encounter, when many may have relocated, some may have died, and some may not want to be reminded about an unpleasant or traumatic experience. There's also evidence that consenters and nonconsenters differ on important characteristics, resulting in potentially biased data sets.[2]

Consent isn't always required to share personal information, of course. A law or regulation could mandate the sharing of personal health information with law enforcement under certain conditions without consent (e.g., the reporting of gunshot wounds) or the reporting of cases of certain infectious diseases without consent (e.g., tuberculosis or HIV).

Sometimes medical staff have fairly broad discretionary authority to share information with public health departments. But not all health care providers are willing to share their patients' personal health information, and many decide not to when it's up to them to decide.[3] So it shouldn't be taken for granted that data custodians would be readily willing to share personal health information, even if they were permitted, and even if it were for the common good.

Anonymization allows for the sharing of health information when it's not mandated or practical to obtain consent, and when the sharing is discretionary and the data custodian doesn't want to share that data.

Penny Pinching

There's actually quite a compelling financial case that can be made for anonymization. The costs from breach notification can be quite high, estimated at $200 per affected individual.[4] For large databases, this adds up to quite a lot of money. However, if the data was anonymized, no breach notification is needed. In this case, anonymization allows you to avoid the costs of a breach response. A recent return-on-investment analysis showed that the expected returns from the anonymization of health data are quite significant, considering just the cost avoidance of breach notification.[5]

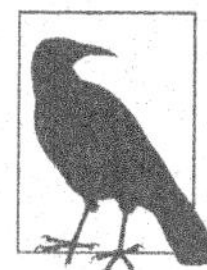

Many jurisdictions have data breach notification laws. This means that whenever there's a data breach involving personal (health) information—such as a lost USB stick, a stolen laptop, or a database being hacked into—there's a need to notify the affected individuals, the media, the attorneys general, or regulators. For example, in the U.S. there are extensive and expensive breach reporting requirements under the Health Insurance Portability and Accountability Act (HIPAA), and 47 states plus D.C. have additional requirements (a handful even require notice if only heatlh data was involved, with no mention of financially relevant information).

Some data custodians make their data recipients subcontractors (these are called Business Associates in the US under HIPAA, and Agents in Ontario under its health privacy law). As subcontractors, these data recipients are permitted to get personal health information under certain circumstances and subject to strict contractual requirements. The subcontractor agreements can make the subcontractor liable for all costs associated with a breach, effectively shifting some of the financial risk to the subcontractors. But even assuming that the subcontractor has a realistic financial capacity to take on such a risk, the data custodian may still suffer indirect costs due to reputational damage and lost business if there is a breach.

Poor anonymization or lack of anonymization can also be costly if individuals are re-identified or re-anonymized (i.e., the reversal of de-identification or anonymization). You may recall the story of AOL, when the company made the search queries of more than half a million of its users publicly available to facilitate research. Soon afterward, *New York Times* reporters were able to re-identify an individual from her search queries. A class action lawsuit was launched and recently settled, with five million dollars going to the class members and one million to the lawyers.[6] Therefore, it's important to have effective and defensible anonymization techniques if data is going to be shared for secondary purposes.

Regulators are also starting to look at anonymization practices during their audits and investigations. In some jurisdictions, such as under HIPAA in the US, the regulator can impose penalties. Recent HIPAA audit findings have identified weaknesses in anonymization practices, so this is clearly one of the factors that they'll be looking at.[7]

People Are Private

We know from surveys of the general public and of patients (adults and youth) that a large percentage of people admit to adopting privacy-protective behaviors because they're concerned about how and for what reasons their health information might be used and disclosed. Privacy-protective behaviors include things like deliberately omitting information from personal or family medical history, self-treating or self-medicating instead of seeking care at a provider, lying to the doctor, paying cash to avoid having a claims record, seeing multiple providers so no individual provider has a complete record, and asking the doctor not to record certain pieces of information.

Youth are mostly concerned about information leaking to their parents, but some are also concerned about future employability. Adults are concerned about insurability and employability, as well as social stigma and the financial and psychological impact of decisions that can be made with their data.

Let's consider a concrete example. Imagine a public health department that gets an Access to Information (or Freedom of Information) request from a newspaper for a database of anonymous test results for a sexually transmitted disease. The newspaper subsequently re-identifies the Mayor of Gotham in that database and writes a story about it. In the future, it's likely that very few people will get tested for that disease, and possibly other sexually transmitted diseases, because they don't trust that the information will stay private. From a public health perspective that's a terrible outcome—the disease is now more likely to be transmitted among more people, and progress to a symptomatic or more severe stage before treatment begins.

The privacy-preserving behaviors we've mentioned are potentially detrimental to patients' health because it makes it harder for the patients to receive the best possible care. It also corrupts the data, because such tactics are the way patients can exercise control over their personal health information. If many patients corrupt their data in subtle ways, then the resultant analytics may not be meaningful because information is missing or incorrect, or the cohorts are incomplete.

Maintaining the public's and patients' trust that their health information is being shared and anonymized responsibly is clearly important.

The Two Pillars of Anonymization

The terminology in this space isn't always clear, and often the same terms are used to mean different, and sometimes conflicting, things.[8] Therefore it's important at the outset to be clear about what we're talking about.

We'll use *anonymization* as an overarching term to refer to everything that we do to protect the identities of individuals in a data set. ISO Technical Specification ISO/TS 25237 (Health informatics—Pseudonymization) provides a good generally accepted definition to use. We then define the two pillars—masking and de-identification—as you can see in Figure 1-1. These are the definitions we use to distinguish between two very different approaches to anonymization.

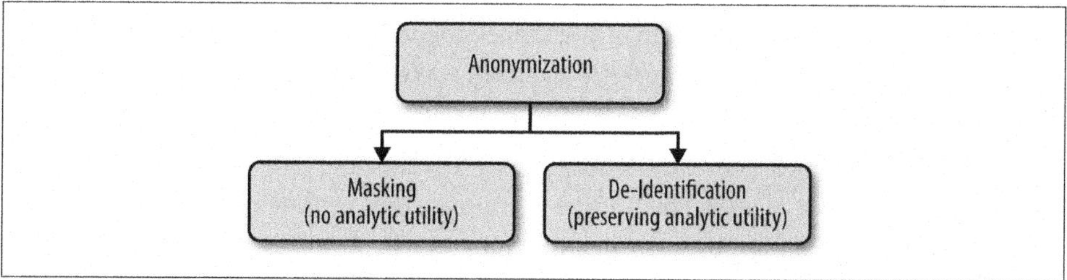

Figure 1-1. The support on which anonymization rests: masking and de-identification.

Anonymization
: A process that removes the association between the identifying data and the data subject (ISO/TS 25237). This is achieved through masking and de-identification.

Masking
: Reducing the risk of identifying a data subject to a very small level by applying a set of data transformation techniques without any concern for the analytic utility of the data.

De-identification
: Reducing the risk of identifying a data subject to a very small level by applying a set of data transformation techniques such that the resulting data retains very high analytic utility.

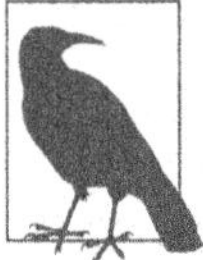

> Masking and de-identification deal with different fields in a data set, so some fields will be masked and some fields will be de-identified. Masking involves protecting things like names and Social Security numbers (SSNs), which are called direct identifiers. De-identification involves protecting fields covering things like demographics and individuals' socioeconomic information, like age, home and work ZIP codes, income, number of children, and race, which are called indirect identifiers.

Masking tends to distort the data significantly so that no analytics can be performed on it. This isn't usually a problem because you normally don't want to perform analytics on the fields that are masked anyway. De-identification involves minimally distorting the data so that meaningful analytics can still be performed on it, while still being able to make credible claims about protecting privacy. Therefore, de-identification involves maintaining a balance between data utility and privacy.

Masking Standards

The only standard that addresses an important element of data masking is ISO Technical Specification 25237. This focuses on the different ways that pseudonyms can be created (e.g., reversible versus irreversible). It doesn't go over specific techniques to use, but we'll illustrate some of these in this book (specifically in Chapter 11).

Another obvious data masking technique is suppression: removing a whole field. This is appropriate in some contexts. For example, if a health data set is being disclosed to a researcher who doesn't need to contact the patients for follow-up questions, there's no need for any names or SSNs. In that case, all of these fields will be removed from the data set. On the other hand, if a data set is being prepared to test a software application, we can't just remove fields because the application needs to have data that matches its database schema. In that case, the names and SSNs are retained but are randomized.

Masking is often interpreted to mean randomization, which involves replacing actual values with random values selected from a large database.[4] You could use a database of first and last names, for example, to randomize those fields. You can also generate random SSNs to replace the original ones. While it may seem easy, if not done well, randomization can still leak personal information or can be easily reversed. For example, *do not* generate a single random number and then add the same number to all SSNs in the data set to "randomize" them.

De-Identification Standards

In general, three approaches to the de-identification of health data have emerged over the last few decades: lists, heuristics, and a risk-based methodology.

Lists

A good example of this approach is the Safe Harbor standard in the HIPAA Privacy Rule. Safe Harbor specifies 18 data elements that need to be removed or generalized (i.e., reducing the precision of the data elements). If you do that to data, that data is considered de-identified according to HIPAA. The Safe Harbor standard was intended to be a simple "cookie cutter" approach that can be applied by any kind of entity covered by HIPAA (a "Covered Entity," or CE). Its application doesn't require much sophistication or knowledge of de-identification methods. However, you need to be cautious about the "actual knowledge" requirement that is also part of Safe Harbor (see the discussion in the sidebar that follows).

The lists approach has been quite influential globally. We know that it has been incorporated into guidelines used by research, government, and commercial organizations in Canada. At the time of writing, the European Medicines Agency was considering such an approach as a minimal standard to de-identify clinical trials data so that it can be shared more broadly.[9]

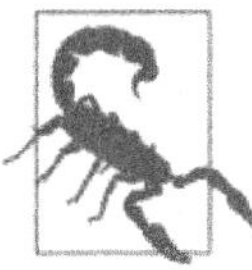

This "list" approach to de-identification has been significantly criticized because it doesn't provide real assurances that there's a low risk of re-identification.[5] It's quite easy to create a data set that meets the Safe Harbor requirements and still have a significantly high risk of re-identification.

What's "Actual Knowledge"?

The HIPAA Privacy Rule Safe Harbor de-identification standard (*http://bit.ly/hipaa-privacy-rule*) includes the requirement that the Covered Entity doesn't have *actual knowledge* that the information could be used alone or in combination with other information to identify an individual who is a subject of the information (a data subject). This requirement seems to be ignored by some organizations that apply Safe Harbor. But it's an important requirement, and failing to observe it can leave a data set identifiable even if the specified 18 elements are removed or generalized.

Actual knowledge has to be specific to the data set and not just general knowledge about what's theoretically possible. This is *clear and direct knowledge* that residual elements could be used to re-identify individuals, and, therefore, that the data isn't truly de-identified.

If there's a record in the data set with an occupation field "Mayor of Gotham," it will be pretty easy to figure out who that individual is. The Covered Entity would have to remove the occupation field to ensure that this kind of information isn't revealed, even though occupation isn't in HIPAA's list of 18 elements. If Richard Greyson is a data recipient and it's known that he has family in the data set, he could use his background knowledge about them to re-identify relatives in the records, so to be anonymized, the information about these relatives would have to be removed or distorted. If Ms. Cobblepot has an unusually large number of children, which was highly publicized in the media because it's rare and unusual, it would be necessary to remove the number of babies from her record in a data set, or remove her entire record.

In all of these examples, the actions taken to de-identify the data would exceed just dealing with the 18 elements identified in Safe Harbor. A Covered Entity wouldn't be able to determine whether any of these examples applied to its data set unless they analyzed the data carefully. Can a Covered Entity deny that it has actual knowledge if it never looks at the data? This is something for the lawyers to decide!

Heuristics

The second approach uses "heuristics," which are essentially rules of thumb that have developed over the years and are used by data custodians to de-identify their data before release. Sometimes these rules of thumb are copied from other organizations that are believed to have some expertise in de-identification. These tend to be more complicated than simple lists and have conditions and exceptions. We've seen all kinds of heuristics, such as never releasing dates of birth, but allowing the release of treatment or visit dates. But there are all kinds of exceptions for certain types of data, such as for rare diseases or certain rural communities with small populations.

While at an abstract level they may make sense, heuristics aren't usually backed up by defensible evidence or metrics. This makes them unsuitable for data custodians that want to manage their re-identification risk in data releases. And the last thing you want is to find yourself justifying evidence-light rules of thumb to a regulator or judge.

Risk-based methodology

This third approach, which is consistent with contemporary standards from regulators and governments, is the approach we present in this book. It's consistent with the "expert determination method" (also known as the "statistical method") in the HIPAA Privacy Rule, as well as recent guidance documents and codes of practice:

- "Guidance Regarding Methods for De-Identification of Protected Health Information in Accordance with the Health Insurance Portability and Accountability Act (HIPAA) Privacy Rule," by the US Department of Health and Human Services

- "Anonymisation: Managing Data Protection Risk Code of Practice," by the UK Information Commissioner's Office
- "'Best Practice' Guidelines for Managing the Disclosure of De-Identified Health Information," by the Canadian Institute for Health Information in collaboration with Canada Health Infoway
- "Statistical Policy Working Paper 22, Report on Statistical Disclosure Limitation Methodology," by the US Federal Committee on Statistical Methodology

We've distilled the key items from these four standards into twelve characteristics that a de-identification methodology needs.[5] Arguably, then, if a methodology meets these twelve criteria, it should be consistent with contemporary standards and guidelines from regulators.

De-identification consists of changes to the data itself, and controls that can be put in place to manage risk. Conceptually, think of de-identification as consisting of dials that can be adjusted to ensure that the risk of re-identification is acceptable. In the next few chapters we'll be discussing these dials in more depth.

De-Identification Myths

A number of myths about de-identification have been circulating in the media and privacy communities for some time. They're myths because they're not supported by credible evidence. We'll summarize some of the important ones here:

Myth: It's possible to re-identify most, if not all, data.

Current evidence strongly suggests that if you de-identify health data using robust methods, the risk of re-identification can be very small. Known examples of re-identification attacks were not performed on data that was properly de-identified.[10] The methods we describe in this book are robust and would ensure that the risk of re-identification is very small.

Myth: Genomic sequences are not identifiable, or are easy to re-identify.

Under certain conditions it's possible to re-identify genomic sequences,[11, 12] and they're very difficult to adequately de-identify using the kinds of methods we describe here. This applies to all kinds of "-omics" data. The types of data sets that we're focusing on in this book consist of clinical, administrative, and survey data. The sharing and analysis of genomic sequences in a privacy-preserving manner requires the use of secure computation techniques, which we'll touch on in a later chapter.

Anonymization in the Wild

You've probably read this far because you're interested in introducing anonymization within your organization, or helping your clients implement anonymization. If that's the case, there are a number of factors that you need to consider about the deployment of anonymization methods.

Organizational Readiness

The successful deployment of anonymization within an organization—whether it's one providing care, a research organization, or a commercial one—requires that organization to be ready. A key indicator of readiness is that the stakeholders believe that they actually need to anonymize their data. Stakeholders include privacy, compliance officer and legal staff in the organization, the individuals responsible for the line of business, and the IT department.

For example, if the organization is a hospital, the line of business may be the pharmacy department that is planning to share its data with researchers. If they don't believe or are not convinced that the data they share needs to be anonymized, or if they've grown comfortable with less mature forms of anonymization, it will be difficult to implement proper anonymization within that organization.

Sometimes stakeholders in the line of business believe that if a data set does not include full names and SSNs, there's no need to do anything else to anonymize it. But as we'll see throughout this book, other pieces of information in a database can reveal the identities of patients even if their names and SSNs are removed, and certainly that's how privacy laws and regulations view the question. Remember that the majority of publicly known successful re-identification attacks were performed on data sets that just had the names, addresses, and SSNs removed.[13]

Also, sometimes these stakeholders are not convinced that they're sharing data for secondary purposes. If data is being shared for the purpose of providing care, patient consent is implied and there's no need to anonymize the data (and actually, anonymizing data in the context of providing care would be a bad idea). Some stakeholders may argue that sharing health data for quality improvement, public health, and analytics around billing are not secondary purposes. Some researchers have also argued that research isn't a secondary purpose. While there may be some merit to their arguments in general, this isn't usually how standards, guidelines, laws, and regulations are written or interpreted.

The IT department is also an important stakeholder because its members will often be responsible for deploying any technology related to anonymization. Believing that anonymization only involves removing or randomizing names in a database (i.e., data masking), IT departments sometimes assign someone to write a few scripts over a couple of days to solve the data sharing problem. As you will see in the remainder of this book, it's just not that simple. Doing anonymization properly is a legal or regulatory requirement, and not getting it right may have significant financial implications for the organization. The IT department needs to be aligned with that view.

Sometimes the organizations most ready for the deployment of proper anonymization are those that have had a recent data breach—although that isn't a recommended method to reach a state of readiness!

Making It Practical

A number of things are required to make anonymization usable in practice. We've found the following points to be quite important, because while theoretical anonymization methods may be elegant, if they don't meet the test of practicality their broad translation into the real world will be challenging:

- The most obvious criterion is that the anonymization methods must have been used in practice. Data custodians are always reassured by knowledge that someone else has tried the methods that they're employing, and that they worked.
- Data users need to be comfortable with the data produced by the anonymization methods being applied. For example, if anonymization distorts the data in ways that are not clear, makes the data analysis more complicated, or limits the type of analysis that the data users can do, they'll resist using anonymized data.
- The anonymization methods must also be understandable by data users. Especially in cases where care or business decisions are going to be made based on the data analysis, having a clear understanding of the anonymization is important. This also affects whether the data users accept the data.
- Anonymization methods that have been scrutinized by peers and regulators are more likely to be adopted. This means that transparency in the exact anonymization methods being used, their justifications, and assumptions made, helps with their adoption within organizations.[i]
- Needless to say, anonymization methods must be consistent with laws and regulations. Methods that would require changes in the law or paradigm shifts in how private information is perceived will not be adopted by data users because they're simply too risky.
- Data custodians want to automate anonymization so that they don't have to bring in external experts to manually anonymize every single data set they need to share. Analytics is becoming an important driver for business, patient care, and patient

i. In some jurisdictions, this is effectively a requirement. For example, the HIPAA expert determination standard for de-identification requires that the techniques used are based on "generally accepted statistical and scientific principles and methods for rendering information not individually identifiable".

safety in many organizations, so using an inefficient process for getting the anonymized data quickly becomes a bottleneck.

Making It Automated

The techniques for anonymizing health data are quite sophisticated, and involve various forms of metrics and optimization algorithms. This means that some form of automation is needed to apply anonymization in practice. This is true of both small and large data sets.

Automation means that it's possible for individuals who are not statisticians or data analysts to anonymize data sets. We still need the data scientists with expertise in anonymization to develop and improve the anonymization algorithms. But once designed, implemented, and automated, these methods should be accessible to a broader and less specialized audience. Let's call them *anonymization professionals.*

Anonymization professionals need to have an understanding of the methods that are being automated, and they need to perform two things: (a) data preparation, and (b) risk assessment. Both of these are described in the remainig chapters. The basic setup is shown in Figure 1-2.

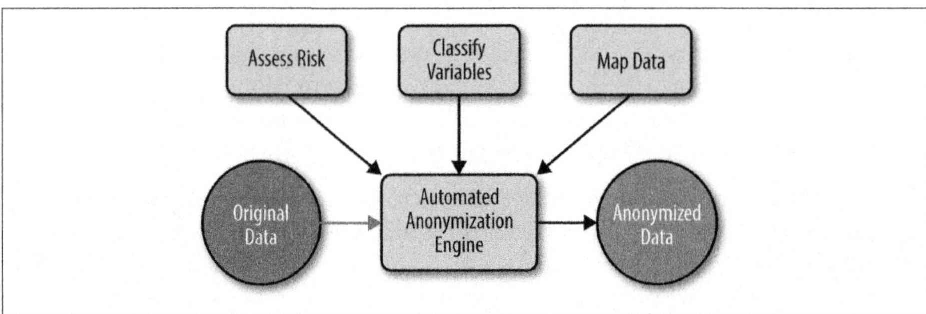

Figure 1-2. The new AA: Automated Anonymization.

The risk assessment step comes down mostly to the completion of a series of checklists that will determine the context of the data release and the context of the re-identification risk. The anonymization professional needs to know the data, the data recipient, and the data custodian well in order to complete the checklist.

The variable classification step includes deciding which variables in the data will be disclosed, and allows an automated system to decide how best to anonymize each variable in the data set. The way each variable is anonymized can be calibrated to the type of variable (e.g., the way a date is anonymized is different from the way a ZIP code is anonymized).

Finally, the data mapping is a technical task that describes how the real data set is organized and the relationships among the tables (assuming a relational data model). For example, a data set may have a table describing the patient demographics and another table describing all of the patient visits. These two tables are linked by a patient ID. All of these details are characterized during the data mapping exercise.

Once these tasks are completed, which an anonymization professional is expected to be able to do, the actual anonymization of a data set can be automated using the techniques described in this book. Simplifying and automating the process in this way reduces the level of technical knowledge needed to anonymize data sets, therefore eliminating the shortage of anonymization professionals. This shortage has been a real obstacle to many data-based research and commercial opportunities.

Use Cases

Practical anonymization has been applied in a number of different situations. The techniques to use will of course depend on the specifics of the situation. Here we summarize some of the use cases:

Research
: This use case is the simplest one, in that the data set can oten be completely defined up front and may not be refreshed or updated. An analyst working for the data custodian decides how to anonymize the data and then creates a file to give to the researcher.

Open data
: There's increasing pressure to make health data openly available on the Web. This may be data from projects funded through the public purse, clinical trials data, or other kinds of government data (so-called "open government" initiatives).

Data warehouses
: Organizations are increasingly creating data warehouses that integrate data sets from multiple sources for the purpose of performing analytics. These sources can be internal to the organization (e.g., different units within the hospital), or external (e.g., data sets from commercial data brokers). Data needs to be anonymized before being pulled out of the data warehouses to perform analytics.

Public health surveillance
: In this use case, health-related data is being continuously collected—from multiple geographically distributed locations—and sent to a centralized database. The sites need to anonymize their data before sending it to the central repository, and the anonymization should be applied consistently across all sites so that the data is meaningful when it is combined. Once the data is collected centrally, it's analyzed and interpreted for things like disease surveillance, evaluating compliance to screening guidelines, and service planning.

Medical devices

Similar to public health surveillance, data from medical devices is collected from multiple sources. The devices themselves can be installed at the sites of health care providers across the country and can pull in data about the patients from electronic medical records. This data could include patient-specific information. Data here is flowing regularly and in many cases needs to be anonymized as it's coming in.

Alerts

This use case is a bit different from the others because an alert needs to be sent close in time to when it was generated. Also, an alert may consist of a very small number of patient records. For example, an alert can be generated for a pharma company when a certain drug is dispensed to a patient. But the information in the alert needs to be de-identified before it can be transmitted. In this case individual (or a small number of) records need to be anonymized on the fly, rather than a full database.

Software testing

This use case often requires access to data to conduct functional and performance tests. Organizations developing applications that process health data need to get that data from production environments. The data from production environments must be anonymized before being sent to the testing group.

We'll discuss many of these use cases in the book and show how they can be handled.

What If the Data Is Re-Identified or De-Anonymized?

A question that often comes up is what would happen if records in a data set that has been properly anonymized were re-identified by an adversary. Assuming that the re-identifications are real and verified, the main concern of the data custodian (or Covered Entity or Business Associate) is whether it is liable. There are a number of things to consider:

- Anonymization is probabilistic—there's a very small probability that records can be re-identified. But it could happen if you're unlucky.
- Zero risk can't guarantee if we want to share any useful data. The very small risk is the trade-off we need to accept to realize the many important benefits of sharing and using health data.
- Regulators don't expect zero risk either—they accept that a very small risk is reasonable.
- There are no court cases or investigations of re-identification attacks by regulators that would set precedents on this issue.
- By following the methods we describe here, you can make a strong case that you are using best contemporary practices, consistent with current standards, guide-

lines, and regulator recommendations. This should help considerably in the case of litigation or investigations.

- Not using defensible methods means that the probability of a successful re-identification attack is much higher (i.e., you are more likely to be unlucky), and the defense you can mount after such an incident would be much weaker.

Therefore, using defensible anonymization methods can reduce risk exposure significantly.

Stigmatizing Analytics

When health data is anonymized so that it can be used for the sake of analytics, the outcome of the analysis is a model or an algorithm. This model can be as simple as a tabular summary of the data, a relationship such as "all people with x have y", a multivariate regression model, or a set of association rules that characterize the relationships in the data. We make a distinction between the process of building this model ("modeling") and making decisions using the model ("decision making").

Anonymized data can be used for modeling. Anonymization addresses the risk of assigning an identity to a record in the database. This promise affects how "personal information" is defined in privacy laws. If the risk of assigning identity is very small, the data will no longer be considered personal information.

Decision making may, however, raise additional privacy concerns. For example, a model could suggest that people living close to an industrial site have a higher incidence of cancer than average making them less employable and reducing their propoerty value. Or a model could be used to send targeted ads to an individual that reveal that that person is gay, pregnant, has had an abortion, or has a mental illness.

In all of these cases, financial, social, and psychological harm may result to the affected individuals. Individuals may be discriminated against due to the decisions made. And in all of these cases the models themselves may have been constructed using anonymized data. The individuals affected by the decisions may not even be in the data sets that were used in building the models. Therefore, opt-out or withdrawal of an individual from a data set wouldn't necessarily have an impact on whether a decision is made about the individual.

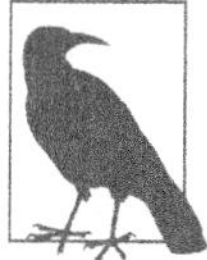

The above are examples of what we call "stigmatizing analytics." These are the types of analytics that produce models that can lead to decisions that adversely affect individuals and groups. Data custodians that anonymize and share health data need to consider the impact of stigmatizing analytics, even though, strictly speaking, it goes beyond anonymization.

The model builders and the decision makers may belong to different organizations. For example, a researcher may build a model from anonymized data and then publish it. Later on, someone else may use the model to make decisions about individual patients.

Data recipients that build models using anonymized health data therefore have another obligation to manage the risks from stigmatizing analytics. In a research context, research ethics boards often play that role, evaluating whether a research study may potentially cause group harm (e.g., to minority groups or groups living in certain geographies) or whether the publication of certain results may stigmatize communities. In such cases they're assessing the conclusions that can be drawn from the resultant models and what kinds of decisions can be made. However, outside the research world, a similar structure needs to be put in place. This governance structure would examine the models and the planned or potential decisions that can be made from the models.

Privacy Ethics

Dealing with stigmatizing analytics is really a question of privacy ethics. Within commercial organizations, one way to manage risks from stigmatizing analytics is to set up a privacy ethics council that would review analytics protocols. This council ought to be somewhat independent because they may have to stop or adjust the development of models or decisions that wouldn't be ethically responsible.

The composition of this council would mirror typical ethics committees. It would have a lay person representing the patients or consumers, a privacy professional, a lawyer, someone representing the business unit, an ethicist, and someone from the public relations department. The last role is important because some analytics protocols may be acceptable or not based only on the reputational or brand harm that it could cause.

The privacy ethics council would advise the business units about the risks from the development of certain models or making certain decisions from models. Having this type of process also ensures that analytics are documented and reviewed before they are included into products and services.

Managing the risks from stigmatizing analytics is an ethical imperative. It can also have a direct impact on patient trust, regulator scrutiny of an organization, and the organization's reputation. Because there is an element of ethics and business impact, social and cultural norms do matter. Some of the factors to consider in this decision-makign include:[14]

- The relationship between the purposes for which the data have been collected and the purposes for further processing.
- The context in which the data have been collected and the reasonable expectations of the data subjects as to their further use.

- The nature of the data and the impact of the further processing on the data subjects.
- The safeguards applied by the controller to ensure fair processing and to prevent any undue impact on the data subjects.

A specific individual or group within the organization should be tasked with reviewing analysis and decision-making protocols to decide whether any fall into the "stigmatizing" category. These individuals should have the requisite backgrounds in ethics, privacy, and business to make the necessary trade-offs and (admittedly), subjective risk assessments.

The fallout from inappropriate models and decisions by data users may go back to the provider of the data. In addition to anonymizing the data they release, data custodians may consider not releasing certain variables to certain data users if there's an increased potential of stigmatizing analytics. They would also be advised to ensure that their data recipients have appropriate mechanisms to manage the risks from stigmatizing analytics.

Anonymization in Other Domains

Although our focus in this book is on health data, many of the methods we describe are applicable to financial, retail, and advertising data. If an online platform needs to report to its advertisers on how many consumers clicked on an ad and segment these individuals by age, location, race, and income, that combination of information may identify some of these individuals with a high probability. The anonymization methods that we discuss here in the context of health data sets can be applied equally well to protect that kind of advertising data.

Basically, the main data fields that make individuals identifiable are similar across these industries: for example, demographic and socioeconomic information. Dates, a very common kind of data in different types of transactions, can also be an identity risk if the transaction is a financial or a retail one. Location is also very important, regardless of domain, both residential and the places they have visited over time. And billing codes might reveal a great deal more than you would expect.

Because of escalating concerns about the sharing of personal information in general, the methods that have been developed to de-identify health data are increasingly being applied in other domains. Additionally, regulators are increasingly expecting the more rigorous methods applied in health care to be more broadly followed in other domains.

Genetics, Cut from a Different Cloth

The methods described in this book aren't suitable for the anonymization of genetic data, and would cause significant distortion to long sequences. The assumptions needed to de-identify sequences of patient events (e.g., visits and claims) would not apply to genomic or other "-omic" data. But there are nuances that are worth considering.

Some of the attacks that have been performed on genomic data didn't actually take advantage of the sequence information at all. In one attack, the dates of birth and ZIP codes that participants included in their profiles for the Personal Genome Project (PGP) were used to re-identify them.[15] This attack used variables that can easily be protected using the techniques we describe in this book. Another attack on PGP exploited the fact that individuals were uploading compressed files that had their names used as filenames when uncompressed.

To the extent that phenotypic information can be inferred from genetic data, such information could possibly be used in a re-identification attack. Predictions (varying in accuracy) of various physical features and certain diagnoses have been reported from genetic information.[16, 17, 18, 19] There have not been any full demonstrations of attacks using this kind of information. Because of the errors in some of these predictions, it's not even clear that they would be useful for a re-identification attack.

More direct attacks are, however, plausible. There is evidence that a sequence of 30 to 80 independent single-nucleotide polymorphisms (SNPs) could uniquely identify a single person.[20] Although such an attack requires the adversary to have genotype data for a target individual, it's also possible to determine whether an individual is in a pool of several thousand SNPs using summary statistics on the proportion of individuals in the case or control group.[11] By utilizing a common Y-chromosome and surname correlation, and relying on generally available recreational genetic genealogy databases, a recent attack was also able to recover individuals' surnames under certain circumstances.[12]

One approach to avoiding these types of attacks is to use secure multiparty computation. This is a set of techniques and protocols that allow sophisticated mathematical and statistical operations to be performed on encrypted data. We look at an example of secure computation in Chapter 12, which focuses on the problem of secure linking. However, the application of these methods to genetic data is still in the early stages of research and we may have to wait a few more years to see some large-scale practical results.

About This Book

Like an onion, this book has layers. Chapter 2 introduces our overall methodology to de-identification (spoiler alert: it's risk-based), including the threats we consider. It's a big chapter, but an important one to read in order to understand the basics of de-identification. Skip it at your own risk!

After that we jump into case studies that highlight the methods we want to demonstrate —from cross-sectional to longitudinal data to more methods to deal with different problems depending on the complexity of the data. The case studies are two-pronged:

they are based on both a method and a type of data. The methods start with the basics, with Chapter 3, then Chapter 4. But longitudinal data can be complicated, given the number of records per patient or the size of the data sets involved. So we keep refining methods in Chapter 5 and Chapter 6. For both cross-sectional and longitudinal data sets, when you want to lighten the load, you may wish to consider the methods of Chapter 7.

For something completely different, and to deal with the inevitable free-form text fields we find in many data sets, we look at text anonymization in Chapter 8. Here we can again measure risk to de-identify, although the methods are very different from what's presented in the previous chapters of the book.

Something else we find in many data sets is the locations of patients and their providers. To anonymize this data, we turn to the geospatial methods in Chapter 9. And we would be remiss if we didn't also include Chapter 10, not only because medical codes are frequently present in health data, but because we get to highlight the Cajun Code Fest (seriously, what a great name).

We mentioned that there are two pillars to anonymization, so inevitably we needed Chapter 11 to discuss masking. We also describe ways to bring data sets together before anonymization with secure linking in Chapter 12. This opens up many new opportunities for building more comprehensive and detailed data sets that otherwise wouldn't be possible. And last but not least, we discuss something on everyone's mind—data quality—in Chapter 13. Obviously there are trade-offs to be made when we strive to protect patient privacy, and a lot depends on the risk thresholds in place. We strive to produce the best quality data we can while managing the risk of re-identification, and ultimately the purpose of this book is to help you balance those competing interests.

References

1. Article 29 Working Party, "Opinion 03/2014 on Purpose Limitation," WP203, Apr. 2013.

2. K. El Emam, E. Jonker, E. Moher, and L. Arbuckle, "A Review of Evidence on Consent Bias in Research," *American Journal of Bioethics* 13:4 (2013): 42–44.

3. K. El Emam, J. Mercer, K. Moreau, I. Grava-Gubins, D. Buckeridge, and E. Jonker. "Physician Privacy Concerns When Disclosing Patient Data for Public Health Purposes During a Pandemic Influenza Outbreak," *BMC Public Health* 11:1 (2011): 454.

4. K. El Emam, *A Guide to the De-identification of Personal Health Information*, (Boca Raton, FL: CRC Press/Auerbach, 2013).

5. *Risky Business: Sharing Health Data While Protecting Privacy*, ed. K. El Emam (Bloomington, IN: Trafford Publishing, 2013).

6. Landweher vs AOL Inc. Case No. 1:11-cv-01014-CMH-TRJ (*http://bit.ly/landweher-vs-AOL*) in the District Court in the Eastern District of Virginia.

7. L. Sanches, "2012 HIPAA Privacy and Security Audits," Office for Civil Rights, Department of Health and Human Services.

8. B. M. Knoppers and M. Saginur "The Babel of Genetic Data Terminology," Nat. Biotechnol., vol. 23, no. 8, pp. 925–927, Aug. 2005.

9. European Medicines Agency, "Publication and access to clinical-trial data," Policy 70, Jun. 2013.

10. K. El Emam, E. Jonker, L. Arbuckle, and B. Malin, "A Systematic Review of Re-Identification Attacks on Health Data," *PLoS ONE* 6:12 (2011): e28071.

11. N. Homer, S. Szelinger, M. Redman, D. Duggan, W. Tembe, J. Muehling, J.V. Pearson, D.A. Stephan, S.F. Nelson, and D.W. Craig, "Resolving Individuals Contributing Trace Amounts of DNA to Highly Complex Mixtures Using High-Density SNP Genotyping Microarrays," *PLoS Genetics* 4:8 (2008): e1000167.

12. M. Gymrek, A.L. McGuire, D. Golan, E. Halperin, and Y. Erlich, "Identifying Personal Genomes by Surname Inference," *Science* 339:6117 (2013): 321–324.

13. K. El Emam, E. Jonker, L. Arbuckle, and B. Malin, "A Systematic Review of Re-Identification Attacks on Health Data," PLoS ONE, vol. 6, no. 12, p. e28071, Dec. 2011.

14. Article 29 Working Party, "Opinion 03/2014 on Purpose Limitation," WP203, Apr. 2013.

15. L. Sweeney, A. Abu, and J. Winn, "Identifying Participants in the Personal Genome Project by Name," (Cambridge, MA: Harvard University, 2013).

16. W. Lowrance and F. Collins, "Identifiability in Genomic Research," *Science* 317:5838 (2007): 600–602.

17. B. Malin and L. Sweeney, "Determining the Identifiability of DNA Database Entries," *Proceedings of the American Medical Informatics Association Annual Symposium*, (Bethesda, MD: AMIA, 2000), 537–541.

18. M. Wjst, "Caught You: Threats to Confidentiality due to the Public Release of Large-scale Genetic Data Sets," *BMC Medical Ethics*, 11:(2010): 21.

19. M. Kayser and P. de Knijff, "Improving Human Forensics Through Advances in Genetics Genomics and Molecular Biology," *Nature Reviews Genetics* 12:(2011): 179–192.

20. Z. Lin, A. Owen, and R. Altman, "Genomic Research and Human Subject Privacy," *Science* 305:(2004): 183.

CHAPTER 2
A Risk-Based De-Identification Methodology

Before we can describe how we de-identified any health data sets, we need to describe some basic methodology. It's a necessary evil, but we'll keep the math to a bare minimum. The complete methodology and its justifications have been provided in detail elsewhere.[1] Here we'll just provide a high-level description of the key steps. The case studies that we go through in subsequent chapters will illustrate how each of these steps applies to real data. This will help you understand in a concrete way how de-identification actually works in practice.

Basic Principles

Some important basic principles guide our methodology for de-identification. These principles are consistent with existing privacy laws in multiple jurisdictions.

The risk of re-identification can be quantified

Having some way to measure risk allows us to decide whether it's too high, and how much de-identification needs to be applied to a data set. This quantification is really just an estimate under certain assumptions. The assumptions concern data quality and the type of attack that an adversary will likely launch on a data set. We start by assuming ideal conditions about data quality for the data set itself and the information that an adversary would use to attack the data set. This assumption, although unrealistic, actually results in conservative estimates of risk (i.e., setting the risk estimate a bit higher than it probably is) because the better the data is, the more likely it is that an adversary will successfully re-identify someone. It's better to err on the conservative side and be protective, rather than permissive, with someone's personal health information. In general, scientific evidence has tended to err on the conservative side—so our reasoning is consistent with some quite strong precedents.

The Goldilocks principle: balancing privacy with data utility

It's important that we produce data sets that are useful. Ideally, we'd like to have a data set that has both maximal privacy protection and maximal usefulness. Unfortunately, this is impossible. Like Goldilocks, we want to fall somewhere in the middle, where privacy is good, but so is data utility. As illustrated in Figure 2-1, maximum privacy protection (i.e., zero risk) means very little to no information being released. De-identification will always result in some loss of information, and hence a reduction in data utility. We want to make sure this loss is minimal so that the data can still be useful for data analysis afterwards. But at the same time we want to make sure that the risk is very small. In other words, we strive for an amount of de-identification that's just right to achieve these two goals.

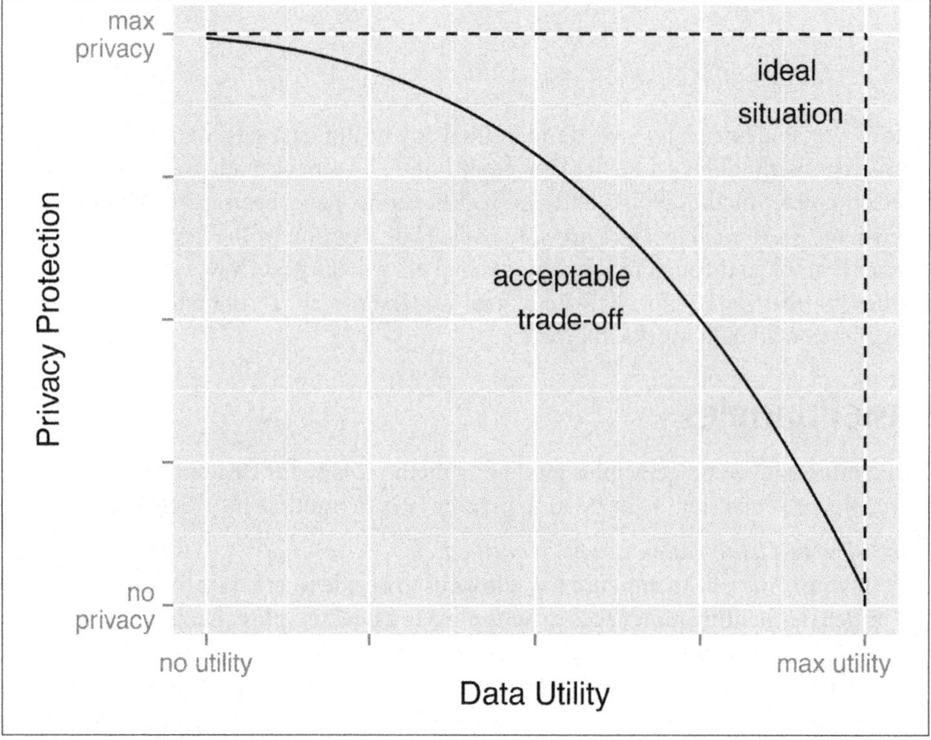

Figure 2-1. The trade-off between perfect data and perfect privacy

The re-identification risk needs to be very small

It's not possible to disclose health data and guarantee zero risk of records being re-identified. Requiring zero risk in our daily lives would mean never leaving the house! What we want is access to data and a *very small* risk of re-identification. It turns out that the definition of *very small* will depend on the context. For example, if we're releasing data on a public website, the definition of *very small* risk is quite different from if we are releasing data to a trusted researcher who has good security and privacy practices in place. A repeatable process is therefore needed to account for this context when defining acceptable risk thresholds.

De-identification involves a mix of technical, contractual, and other measures
: A number of different approaches can be used to ensure that the risk of re-identification is very small. Some techniques can be contractual, some can be related to proper governance and oversight, and others can be technical, requiring modifications to the data itself. In practice, a combination of these approaches is used. It's considered reasonable to combine a contractual approach with a technical approach to get the overall risk to be very small. The point is that it's not necessary to use only a technical approach.

Steps in the De-Identification Methodology

There are some basic tasks you'll have to perform on a data set to achieve the degree of de-identification that's acceptable for your purposes. Much of the book will provide detailed techniques for carrying out these steps.

Step 1: Selecting Direct and Indirect Identifiers

The *direct identifiers* in a data set are those fields that can essentially be used alone to uniquely identify individuals or their households. An individual's Social Security number is considered a direct identifier, because there's only one person with that number. A person's name is also considered a direct identifier, because many names are unique (take ours as examples!), particularly in a single data set.

Indirect identifiers are other fields in the data set that can be used in combination with one another to identify individuals. For example, date of birth and geographic location, such as a ZIP or postal code, are considered indirect identifiers. There may be more than one person with the same birthdate in your ZIP code, but maybe not! And the more indirect identifiers you have, the more likely it becomes that an attacker can pinpoint an individual in the data set. Indirect identifiers are also referred to as *quasi-identifiers* in the computational disclosure control literature, and as *key variables* in the statistical disclosure control literature. They all mean the same thing.

Examples of Direct and Indirect Identifiers

Examples of direct identifiers include name, telephone number, fax number, email address, health insurance card number, credit card number, Social Security number, medical record number, and social insurance number.

Examples of indirect or quasi-identifiers include sex, date of birth or age, location (such as postal code, census geography, and information about proximity to known or unique landmarks), language spoken at home, ethnic origin, aboriginal identity, total years of schooling, marital status, criminal history, total income, visible minority status, activity difficulties/reductions, profession, event dates (such as dates of admission, discharge, procedure, death, specimen collection, or visit/encounter), codes (such as diagnosis codes, procedure codes, and adverse event codes), country of birth, birth weight, and birth plurality.

Identifiers must be replicable, distinguishable, and knowable.[2] A field in a data set is replicable if its values are stable over time. Blood sugar level will vary considerably and therefore would not be a good identifier. A field is distinguishable if it has sufficient variation to distinguish among inidviduals in the data set. The diagnosis of breast cancer in a breast cancer database is not distinguishable, although secondary diagnoses would be.

Both types of identifying fields, direct or indirect, must characterize information that an adversary can know and then use to re-identify the records in the data set, i.e., they must be knowable. The adversaries might know this information because they're acquaintances of individuals in the data set (e.g., relatives or neighbors), or because that information exists in a public registry (e.g., a voter registration list). The distinction between these two types of fields is important because the method you'll use for anonymization will depend strongly on such distinctions. A decison tree summarizing the steps is provided in Figure 2-2.

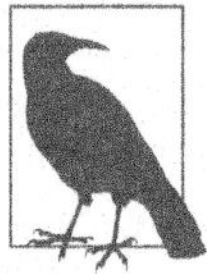

We use masking techniques to anonymize the direct identifiers, and de-identification techniques to anonymize the quasi-identifiers. If you're not sure whether a field is a direct or quasi- identifier, and it will be used in a statistical analysis, then treat it as a quasi-identifier. Otherwise you lose that information entirely, because masking doesn't produce fields that are useful for analytics, whereas a major objective of de-identifying indirect identifiers is to preserve analytic integrity (as described in "Step 4: De-Identifying the Data" on page 28).

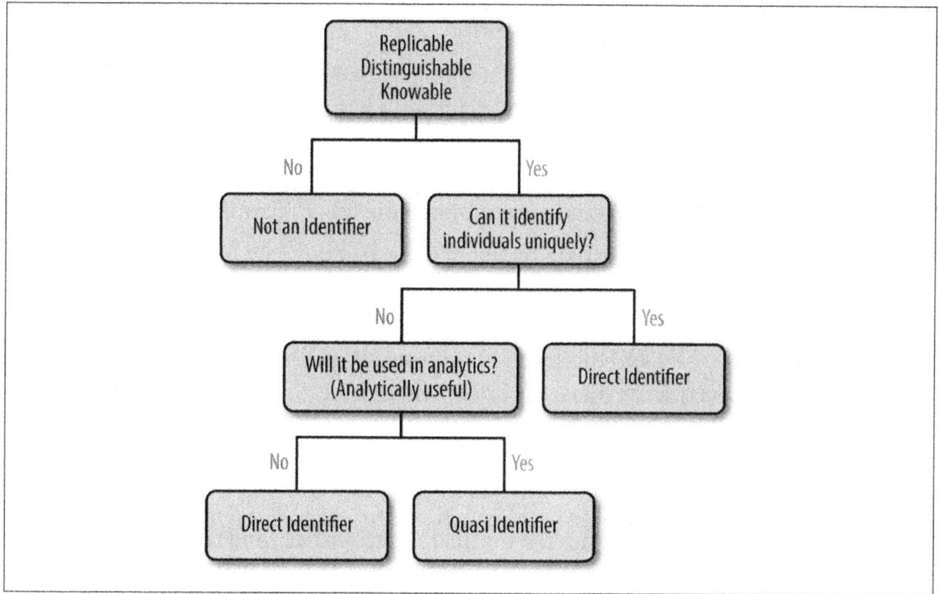

Figure 2-2. The tree of (anonymization) life, to help you decide if a field is an identifier or not, and if so then of which type.

Step 2: Setting the Threshold

The risk threshold represents the maximum acceptable risk for sharing the data. This threshold needs to be quantitative and defensible. There are two key factors to consider when setting the threshold:

- Is the data going to be in the public domain (a public use file, for example)?
- What's the extent of the *invasion of privacy* when this data is shared as intended?

A public data set has no restrictions on who has access to it or what users can do with it. For example, a data set that will be posted on the Internet, as part of an open data or an open government initiative, would be considered a public data set. For a data set that's not going to be publicly available, you'll know who the data recipient is and can impose certain restrictions and controls on that recipient (more on that later).

The invasion of privacy evaluation considers whether the data release would be considered an invasion of the privacy of the data subjects. Things that we consider include the sensitivity of the data, potential harm to patients in the event of an inadvertent disclosure, and what consent mechanisms existed when the data was originally collected (e.g., did the patients consent to this use or disclosure?). We've developed a detailed checklist for assessing and scoring invasion of privacy elsewhere.[1]

Step 3: Examining Plausible Attacks

Four plausible attacks can be made on a data set. The first three are relevant when there's a known data recipient, and the last is relevant only to public data sets:

1. The data recipient deliberately attempts to re-identify the data.
2. The data recipient inadvertently (or spontaneously) re-identifies the data.
3. There's a data breach at the data recipient's site and the data is "in the wild."
4. An adversary can launch a demonstration attack on the data.

If the data set will be used and disclosed by a known data recipient, then the first three attacks need to be considered plausible ones. These three cover the universe of attacks we've seen empirically. There are two general factors that affect the probability of these three types of attacks occurring:

Motives and capacity
: Whether the data recipient has the motivation, resources, and technical capacity to re-identify the data set

Mitigating controls
: The security and privacy practices of the data recipient

We've developed detailed checklists for assessing and scoring these factors elsewhere.[1]

Motives can be managed by having enforceable contracts with the data recipient. Such an agreement will determine how likely a deliberate re-identification attempt would be.

Managing the Motives of Re-Identification

It's important to manage the motives of re-identification for data recipients. You do that by having contracts in place, and these contracts need to include very specific clauses:

- A prohibition on re-identification
- A requirement to pass on that prohibition to any other party the data is subsequently shared with
- A prohibition on attempting to contact any of the patients in the data set
- An audit requirement that allows you to conduct spot checks to ensure compliance with the agreement, or a requirement for regular third-party audits

Without such a contract, there are some very legitimate ways to re-identify a data set. Consider a pharmacy that sells prescription data to a consumer health portal. The data is de-identified using the HIPAA Safe Harbor de-identification standard (*http://bit.ly/hipaa-privacy-rule*) and contains patient age, gender, dispensed drug information, the pharmacy location, and all of the physician details (we've discussed the privacy of prescription data elsewhere).[3,4] So, in the eyes of HIPAA there are now few restrictions on that data.

The portal operator then matches the prescription data from the pharmacy with other data collected through the portal to augment the patient profiles. How can the portal do that? Here are some ways:

- The prescriber is very likely the patient's doctor, so the data will match that way.
- Say the portal gets data from the pharmacy every month. By knowing when a data file is received, the portal will know that the prescription was dispensed in the last month, even if the date of the prescription is not provided as part of the data set.
- The patient likely lives close to the prescriber—so the portal would look for patients living within a certain radius of the prescriber.
- The patient likely lives close to the pharmacy where the drug was dispensed—so the portal would also look for patients living within a certain radius of the pharmacy.
- The portal can also match on age and gender.

With the above pieces of information, the portal can then add to the patients' profiles with their exact prescription information and deliver competing drug advertisements when patients visit the portal. This is an example of a completely legitimate re-identification attack on a data set that uses Safe Harbor. Unless there is a contract with the pharmacy explicitly prohibiting such a re-identification, there is nothing keeping the portal from doing this.

Mitigating controls will have an impact on the likelihood of a rogue employee at the data recipient being able to re-identify the data set. A rogue employee may not necessarily be bound by a contract unless there are strong mitigating controls in place at the data recipient's site.

A demonstration attack, the fourth in our list of attacks, occurs when an adversary wants to make a point of showing that a data set can be re-identified. The adversary is not looking for a specific person, but the one or more that are easiest to re-identify—it is an attack on low-hanging fruit. It's the worst kind of attack, producing the highest probability of re-identification. A demonstration attack has some important features:

- It requires only a single record to be re-identified to make the point.
- Because academics and the media have performed almost all known demonstration attacks,[5] the available resources to perform the attack are usually scarce (i.e., limited money).

- Publicizing the attack is important for the success of its aspects as a demonstration, so illegal or suspect behaviors will not likely be performed as part of the attack (e.g., using stolen data or misrepresentation to get access to registries).

The first of these features can lead to an overestimation of the risks in the data set (remember, no data set is guaranteed to be free of re-identification risk). But the latter two features usually limit the why and how to a smaller pool of adversaries, and point to ways that we can reduce their interest in re-identifying a record in a data set (e.g., by making sure that the probability of success is sufficiently low that it would exhaust their resources). There's even a manifesto for privacy researchers on ethically launching a demonstration attack.[6] Just the same, if a data set will be made publicly available, without restrictions, then this is the worst case that must be considered because the risk of an attack on low-hanging fruit is, in general, possible.

In a public data release our only defense against re-identification is modifying the data set. There are no other controls we can use to manage re-identification risk, and the Internet has a long memory. Unfortunately, this will result in a data set that has been modified quite a bit. When disclosing data to a known data recipient, other controls can be put in place, such as the contract and security and privacy practice requirements in that contract. These additional controls will reduce the overall risk and allow fewer modifications to the data.

The probabilities of these four types of attacks can be estimated in a reasonable way, as we'll describe in "Probability Metrics" on page 33, allowing you to analyze the actual overall risk of each case. For a nonpublic data set, if all of the three risk values for attacks 2–4 are below the threshold determined in "Step 2: Setting the Threshold" on page 25, the overall re-identification risk can be considered very small.

Step 4: De-Identifying the Data

The actual process of de-identifying a data set involves applying one or more of three different techniques:

Generalization
: Reducing the precision of a field. For example, the date of birth or date of a visit can be generalized to a month and year, to a year, or to a five-year interval. Generalization maintains the truthfulness of the data.

Suppression
: Replacing a value in a data set with a NULL value (or whatever the data set uses to indicate a missing value). For example, in a birth registry, a 55-year-old mother would have a high probability of being unique. To protect her we would suppress her age value.

Subsampling
: Releasing only a simple random sample of the data set rather than the whole data set. For example, a 50% sample of the data may be released instead of all of the records.

These techniques have been applied extensively in health care settings and we've found them to be acceptable to data analysts. They aren't the only techniques that have been developed for de-identifying data, but many of the other ones have serious disadvantages. For example, data analysts are often very reluctant to work with synthetic data, especially in a health care context. The addition of noise can often be reversed using various filtering methods. New models, like differential privacy, have some important practical limitations that make them unsuitable, at least for applications in health care.[7] And other techniques have not been applied extensively in health care settings, so we don't yet know if or how well they work.

Step 5: Documenting the Process

From a regulatory perspective, it's important to document the process that was used to de-identify the data set, as well as the results of enacting that process. The process documentation would be something like this book or a detailed methodology text.[1] The results documentation would normally include a summary of the data set that was used to perform the risk assessment, the risk thresholds that were used and their justifications, assumptions that were made, and evidence that the re-identification risk after the data has been de-identified is below the specified thresholds.

Measuring Risk Under Plausible Attacks

To measure re-identification risk in a meaningful way, we need to define plausible attacks. The metrics themselves consist of probabilities and conditional probabilities. We won't go into detailed equations, but we will provide some basic concepts to help you understand how to capture the context of a data release when deciding on plausible attacks. You'll see many examples of these concepts operationalized in the rest of the book.

T1: Deliberate Attempt at Re-Identification

Most of the attacks in this section take place in a relatively safe environment, where the institution we give our data to promises to keep it private. Consider a situation where we're releasing a data set to a researcher. That researcher's institution, say a university, has signed a data use agreement that prohibits re-identification attempts. We can assume that as a legal entity the university will comply with the contracts that it signs. We can then say that the university does not have the motivation to re-identify the data. The university may have some technical capacity to launch a re-identification attack, though. These two considerations make up the dimension of *motives and capacity*.

Our assumptions can't rule out the possibility that someone at the university will deliberately attempt to re-identify the data. There may be a rogue staff member who wants to monetize the data for personal financial gain. In that case, the probability of a re-identification attack will depend on the controls that the university has in place to manage the data (the dimension of *mitigating controls*).

These two dimensions affect the *Pr*(re-id, attempt) factor of the following equation, which is the probability that the university or its staff will both attempt to and successfully re-identify the data. Assuming now that an attempt will occur, we can then measure the probability that an adversary will successfully re-identify a record. We call the overall probability of re-identification under this scenario attack T1:

Attack T1

$$Pr(\text{re-id, attempt}) = Pr(\text{attempt}) \times Pr(\text{re-id} \mid \text{attempt})$$

The first factor on the righthand side, the probability of attempt, captures the context of the data release; the second factor on the righthand side, the probability of re-identification given an attempt,[i] captures the probability of an adversary actually re-identifying a record in the data set. Each probability is a value between 0.0 and 1.0, so their product will also be in that range.

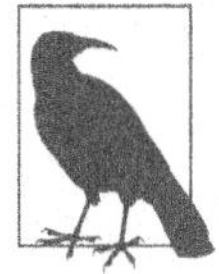

The value of *Pr*(attempt) needs to be estimated based on common sense and experience. It's a subjective estimate that's derived from expert opinion. One scheme for estimating that value has been described elsewhere.[1] The key characteristics of that scheme are that it's conservative—in that it errs on the side of assigning a higher probability to an attempted re-identification even if the data recipient has good controls in place—and it gives results that are consistent with the levels of risk that people have been releasing data with, today and historically.

Another scheme is to say that if *motives and capacity* are managed, then we need to focus on the possibility of a rogue employee. If the data set will be accessed by, say, 100 people, how many rogue employees will there be? If there is likely to be only one rogue employee, then we can say that *Pr*(attempt) is 1/100. If we want to be conservative we can say that 10 of these employees may go rogue—so *Pr*(attempt) = 0.1.

Going back to our example, if the university doesn't sign a data use agreement, or if the agreement doesn't have a prohibition on re-identification attempts by the university,

i. The conditional probability *Pr*(A | B) is read as the probability of A given B, or the probability that A will occur on the condition that B occurs.

the value for *Pr*(attempt) will be high. These types of conditions are taken into account when assessing the *motives and capacity*.

The value of *Pr*(re-id | attempt), which is the probability of correctly re-identifying a record given that an attempt was made, is computed directly from the data set. Specific metrics come later, in "Probability Metrics" on page 33.

T2: Inadvertent Attempt at Re-Identification

Now let's consider the second attack, T2. Under this attack, a staff member at the university inadvertently recognizes someone in the data set. This can be, for example, a data analyst who is working with the data set. The data analyst may recognize an acquaintance, such as a neighbor or a relative, in the data set through the individual's age and ZIP code. Attack T2 is represented as:

Attack T2

$$Pr(\text{re-id, acquaintance}) = Pr(\text{acquaintance}) \times Pr(\text{re-id} \mid \text{acquaintance})$$

The value of *Pr*(acquaintance) captures the probability that that staff member can know someone who is potentially in the data set. For example, if the data set is of breast cancer patients, this probability is that of a randomly selected member of the population knowing someone who has breast cancer. This probability can be computed in a straightforward manner by considering that on average people tend to have 150 friends. This is called the *Dunbar number*. While the exact value for the Dunbar number shows that it varies around 150, it's been consistently shown to be close to 150 for offline and online relationships together.[1] We can also get the prevalence of breast cancer in the population using public data sets. Knowing the prevalence, ρ, and the Dunbar number, we can use the estimate $Pr(\text{acquaintance}) = 1-(1-\rho)^{150/2}$ (we divide the number of friends in half seeing as breast cancer is a disease that predominantly affects women).

If we're considering a data set of breast cancer patients living in California and the adversary is in Chicago, we're only interested in the prevalence of breast cancer in California, not in Chicago. Therefore, the prevalence needs to be specific to the geography of the data subjects. We can assume that the prevalence is more or less the same in California as it is nationally, and use the national number, or we can look up the prevalence for California in order to be more accurate. We wouldn't know if the adversary has 150 acquaintances in California, but we can make the worst-case assumption and say that he does. If the prevalence can't be found, then as a last resort it can be estimated from the data itself. These assumptions would have to be documented.

The next factor in this equation—*Pr*(re-id | acquaintance), the probability of correctly re-identifying a record given that the adversary knows someone in the population covered by the data set—is computed from the data itself. There will be more on that in "Probability Metrics" on page 33.

T3: Data Breach

The third attack, T3, can take place if the university loses the data set—in other words, in the case of a data breach, which was the attack described in "Step 3: Examining Plausible Attacks" on page 26. Current evidence suggests that most breaches occur through losses or thefts of mobile devices. But other breach vectors are also possible. Based on recent credible evidence, we know that approximately 27% of providers that are supposed to follow the HIPAA Security Rule (*http://bit.ly/hipaa-security-rule*) have a reportable breach every year. The HIPAA Security Rule is really a basic set of security practices that an organization needs to have in place—it's a minimum standard only. Attack T3 is represented as:

Attack T3

$$Pr(\text{re-id, breach}) = Pr(\text{breach}) \times Pr(\text{re-id} \mid \text{breach})$$

It should be noted that the 27% breach rate, or $Pr(\text{breach}) = 0.27$, is likely to change over time. But at the time of writing, this is arguably a reasonable estimate of the risk. As with attacks T1 and T2, $Pr(\text{re-id} \mid \text{breach})$ is computed from the data itself, which we cover in "Probability Metrics" on page 33.

Implementing the HIPAA Security Rule

There are a bunch of mitigating controls that need to be considered in dealing with personal health information.[8] These are considered the most basic forms of controls. Think of them as minimum standards only! We can give you only a taste of what's expected, because it's pretty detailed (although this summary covers a lot of ground):

Controlling access, disclosure, retention, and disposition of personal data
: It should go without saying (but we'll say it anyway) that only authorized staff should have access to data, and only when they need it to do their jobs. There should also be data sharing agreements in place with collaborators and subcontractors, and all of the above should have to sign nondisclosure or confidentiality agreements. Of course, data can't be kept forever, so there should also be a data retention policy with limits on long-term use, and regular purging of data so it's not sitting around waiting for a breach to occur. If any data is going to leave the US, there should also be enforceable data sharing agreements and policies in place to control disclosure to third parties.

Safeguarding personal data
: It's important to respond to complaints or incidents, and that all staff receive privacy, confidentiality, and security training. Sanctions are usually doled out to anyone that steps out of line with these policies and procedures, and there's a protocol for privacy breaches that has been put to good use. Authentication measures must be in place with logs that can be used to investigate an incident. Data can be accessed remotely, but that access must be secure and logged. On the technical side, a regularly updated program needs to be in place to prevent malicious or mobile code from being run

on servers, workstations and mobile devices, and data should be transmitted securely. It's also necessary to have physical security in place to protect access to computers and files, with mandatory photo ID.

Ensuring accountability and transparency in the management of personal data
: There needs to be someone senior accountable for the privacy, confidentiality, and security of data, and there needs to be a way to contact that person. Internal or external auditing and monitoring mechanisms also need to be in place.

T4: Public Data

The final attack we consider, T4, is when data is disclosed publicly. In that case we assume that there is an adversary who has background information that can be used to launch an attack on the data, and that the adversary will attempt a re-identification attack. We therefore only consider the probability of re-identification from the data set:

Attack T4
: *Pr*(re-id), based on data set only

So, if we know who, specifically, is getting the data set, we de-identify our data set in the face of assumed attacks T1, T2, and T3; if we don't know who is getting the data set, as in a public data release, we de-identify our data set assuming attack T4.

Measuring Re-Identification Risk

A recent text provided a detailed review of various metrics that can be used to measure re-identification risk.[1] We'll focus on the key risk metrics that we use in our case studies, and explain how to interpret them.

Probability Metrics

When we release a data set, we can assign a probability of re-identification to every single record. To manage the risk of re-identification, however, we need to assign an overall probability value to the whole data set. This allows us to decide whether the whole data set has an acceptable risk. There are two general approaches that we can use: *maximum risk* and *average risk*.

With the maximum risk approach, we assign the overall risk to the record that has the highest probability of re-identification. This is, admittedly, a conservative approach. The key assumption is that the adversary is attempting to re-identify a single person in the data set, and that the adversary will look for the target record that has the highest probability of being re-identified. For instance, the adversary will try to re-identify the record that's the most extreme outlier because that record is likely to be unique in the population. This assumption is valid under attack T4, where we assume a demonstration attack is attempted.

Attack T1 would be a breach of contract, so an adversary is not likely to want to promote or advertise the attempted re-identification. The most likely scenarios are that the adversary is trying to re-identify someone she knows (i.e., a specific target, maybe a friend or relative, or someone famous), or the adversary is trying to re-identify everyone in the data set.

If the adversary is trying to re-identify an acquaintance, any one of the records can be the target, so it's fair to use a form of average risk. This risk is also called *journalist* or *prosecutor risk*, for obvious reasons. If the adversary is trying to re-identify everyone in the data set, it's also a form of average risk, but it's called *marketer risk*. Journalist or prosecutor risk is always greater than or equal to marketer risk, so we only need to focus on journalist or prosecutor risk to manage both scenarios.[1]

In the case of attack T2, a spontaneous recognition ("Holly Smokes, that's my neighbor!"), we follow the same logic. Since we're talking about the re-identification of a single record, but every record is potentially at risk, we again consider the average risk. It's a question of who, on average, might recognize someone they know in the data set.

Finally, for attack T3, we assume that anyone who gets their hands on a breached data set realizes that using it in any way whatsoever is probably illegal. It's therefore pretty unlikely that they would launch a targeted demonstration attack. If they do anything besides report having found the lost data, they won't want to advertise it. So again we can use average risk, because anyone or everyone might be at risk for re-identification.

For each attack, we estimate the same *Pr*(re-id | T) from the data itself, where T is any one of attempt, acquaintance, or breach. In other words, we assume that there is a deliberate attempt, or that there is an acquaintance, or that there is a breach, and treat each of these conditional probabilities as the same. What we've done is operationalize the original concept of *Pr*(re-id, attempt) so that it considers three different forms of "attempts." And we use this to ensure that data sets are less than the re-identification risk threshold, regardless of the form of the attempt.

What's the Data Worth?

If a malicious adversary gets his hands on a data set, what's a single re-identified record worth (e.g., for identify theft)? Not much, apparently. Full identities have been estimated to be worth only \$1–\$15.[9] In one case where hackers broke into a database of prescription records, the ransom amount worked out to only \$1.20 per patient.[10]. In the UK, a hospital outsourced the computerization of its medical records to India and hundreds of records later appeared for sale on the black market for £4 each.[11] If a data set is de-identified, it hardly seems worth the effort to re-identify a single record.

On the other hand, the data set as a whole may be of value if the adversary can ransom it off or sell it. The hackers mentioned above demanded \$10 million from the Virginia Department of Health Professionals. This database was intended to allow pharmacists and health care professionals to track prescription drug abuse, such as incidents of patients who go "doctor-shopping" to find more than one doctor to prescribe narcotics.

In a different case, hackers threatened to publicize the personal information of clients of Express Scripts,[12] a company that manages pharmacy benefits. The company was using production data containing personal information for software testing, and there was a breach on the testing side of the business. Unfortunately, using production data for testing is common. The initial extortion attempt was based on the breach of 75 records. It turned out later that 700,000 individuals might have been affected by the breach.

The problem with average risk is that it allows records that are unique to be released. For example, say we have a data set with a record about Fred, a 99-year-old man living in a particular ZIP code. If Fred is the only 99-year-old in that ZIP code, and this is captured in the data set, it's pretty easy for anyone that knows Fred to re-identify his health records. Worse, assume he's the only male over 90 in that ZIP code; then it's even easier for someone to re-identify his records, perhaps from the voter registration list. It's perfectly reasonable to assume that the average risk for that data set would be quite low because very few records in the data set stand out. So we can release the data set—but what about Fred?

We therefore need a more stringent definition of average risk; one that takes uniques into account. Let's call it *strict average risk*. This is a two-step risk metric:

1. We need to make sure that the maximum risk is below a specific threshold, say 0.5 (i.e., at least two records match) or preferably 0.33 (i.e., at least three records match). Meeting this threshold means getting rid of unique records in the data set, like Fred, through de-identification.
2. Then we evaluate average risk. If the maximum risk in the first step is above the threshold of 0.5 or 0.33, that would be the risk level for the data set. Otherwise, if the maximum risk in the first step is below the threshold, the risk level for the data set is the regular average risk.

Adhering to *strict average risk* ensures that there are no unique individuals in the data set, and is consistent with best practices in the disclosure control community. It keeps the Freds safe!

Information Loss Metrics

When de-identifying a data set, we inevitably lose information (e.g., through generalization or suppression). Information loss metrics give us a concrete way of evaluating the distortion that has been applied to a data set. Ideal information loss metrics would evaluate the extent to which the analytics results change before and after de-identification. But that's not generally practical because it requires precise knowledge of the analytics that will be run before the de-identification can even be applied. What we need are more general information loss metrics.

A lot of these metrics have been cooked up in the academic literature. We've found two that in practice give us the most useful information:

Entropy
: A measure of uncertainty. In our context it reflects the amount of precision lost in the data and can account for changes due to generalization, suppression, and sub-sampling.[13] The greater the entropy, the more the information loss. Pretty straightforward. Even though entropy is a unitless measure, by definition, it can be converted to a percentage by defining the denominator as the maximum possible entropy for a data set. This makes changes in entropy, before and after de-identification, clearer.

Missingness
: A measure of cells or records that are missing. Again straightforward, and an important measure in its own right. High amounts of missingness can reduce the statistical power in a data set, because some records may have to be dropped. And bias can be introduced if missing values are not random. If we take a simple example of a single quasi-identifier, rare and extreme values are more likely to be suppressed for the sake of de-identification. Therefore, by definition, the pattern of suppression will not be completely random.

These two metrics show us different perspectives on information loss. As we use it here, entropy is affected only by the generalizations that are applied. So it gives a measure of how much information was lost due to the generalization that was applied during de-idenitfication. Missingness is affected only by suppression. Therefore, the combination of these two metrics gives us an overall picture of information loss.

The Impact of Missingness

A common way to deal with missing cells in data analysis is Complete Case Analysis (CCA), which simply ignores records with any missingness whatsoever, even in variables that are not included in an analysis. It's the quick and dirty way to get rid of missingness. It's also the default in many statistical packages, and is common practice in epidemiology. But it's pretty well known that this approach to data analysis will result in a hefty loss of data. For example, with only 2% of the values missing at random in each of 10 variables, you would lose 18.3% of the observations on average. With five variables having 10% of their values missing at random, 41% of the observations would be lost on average.[14]

Another common way to deal with missing cells in a data set is Available Case Analysis (ACA), which uses records with complete values for the variables used in a particular analysis. It's much more careful to include as much data as possible, unlike the brute force approach of CCA. For example, in constructing a correlation matrix, different records are used for each pair of variables depending on the availability of both values, but this can produce nonsense results.[14]

Both CCA and ACA are only fully justified under the strong assumption that missingness is completely at random.[15, 16] And suppression done for the sake of de-identification can't be considered random. Of course, most (if not all) missingness in real data is not completely at random either—it's a theoretical ideal. As a result, the amount of suppression, leading to increased missingness, is an important indicator of the amount of distortion caused to the data by the de-identification algorithm.

Our aim is to minimize missingness as much as possible. Of course, you can always collect more data to compensate for loss of statistical power, but that means time and money. When the type of bias is well understood, it's possible to use model-based imputation to recover the missing values (a technique for estimating the missing values through techniques such as averaging the surrounding values or filling in common values). But it's not always possible to create accurate models, and this also adds to the complexity of the analysis.

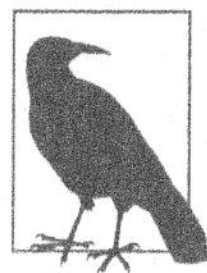

We should clarify that missingness can have two interpretations. It could be the percentage of *records* (rows) that have had any suppression applied to them on any of the quasi-identifiers, or it could be the percentage of *cells* (row and column entries) in the quasi-identifiers that have had some suppression applied to them.

Let's say we have a data set of 100 records and two quasi-identifiers. Three records have "natural" missingness, due to data collection errors, on the first quasi-identifier. These are records 3, 5, and 7. So we have 3 records out of 100 that have missing values, or 3% record missingness. Let's say that de-identification adds some suppression to the second quasi-identifier in records 5, 10, and 18 (i.e., not the same quasi-identifier). In this case, only 2 new records had suppression applied to them due to de-identification (records 10 and 18), so we now have 5 records out of 100 with missing values, or 5% record missingness. Therefore, the information loss is 2% record missingness.

Now consider the second type of missingness, based on the percentage of suppressed cells that are for quasi-identifiers. Our previous example started with 3 missing cells out of 200 (100 cells per quasi-identifier), or 1.5% cell missingness. After de-identification, we had 6 missing cells out of 200, or 3% cell missingness. Therefore, the information loss is 1.5% cell missingness.

Risk Thresholds

We've covered our methodology and how to measure risk, but we also need to discuss the practical aspects of choosing, and meeting, risk thresholds.

Choosing Thresholds

"Measuring Risk Under Plausible Attacks" on page 29 presented four attacks with four equations. What's the maximum acceptable probability of re-identification for the whole data set? It's reasonable to set the same risk threshold for all four attacks, because a patient or regulator won't care which type of attack reveals an identity.

What If a Data Subject Self-Reveals?

There's a lot of interest in making data from academic and industry-sponsored clinical trials more generally available, including having the data made publicly available. But participants in a clinical trial can self-reveal that they're part of such a trial, maybe through their posts to an online social network.

If a data subject self-reveals, that subject's records have a higher probability of being re-identified. This applies whether we use average or maximum risk. Re-identification of a record may reveal additional information about the data subject, such as co-morbidities, other drugs she may be taking, or sensitive information about her functioning or mental well-being.

Because there's a risk of at least one participant in a clinical trial self-revealing that she has participated, should we assume a higher risk for all data subjects in the database? In general, that would be a very conservative approach. There needs to be evidence that many participants in the trial are likely to self-reveal before it would be reasonable to assume an elevated risk of re-identification.

As a cautionary measure, however, it would be important to inform participants in the clinical trial that there is a plan to share trial data broadly, and explain the risks from self-revealing. If participants have been informed of these risks, then arguably it's reasonable to leave the risk as is; if participants have not been informed of these risks, then it may be more prudent to assume an elevated risk.

There are many precedents going back multiple decades for what is an acceptable probability of releasing personal information.[1] The values from these precedents, shown in Figure 2-3, have not changed recently and remain in wide use. In fact, they are recommended by regulators and in court cases. However, all of these precedents are for maximum risk.

As the precedents indicate, when data has been released publicly, the thresholds range between 0.09 and 0.05 for maximum risk. Therefore, it's relatively straightforward to define a threshold for attack T4, where we assume there is the risk of a demonstration attack. If we choose the lowest threshold, we can set the condition that $Pr(\text{re-id}) \leq 0.05$.

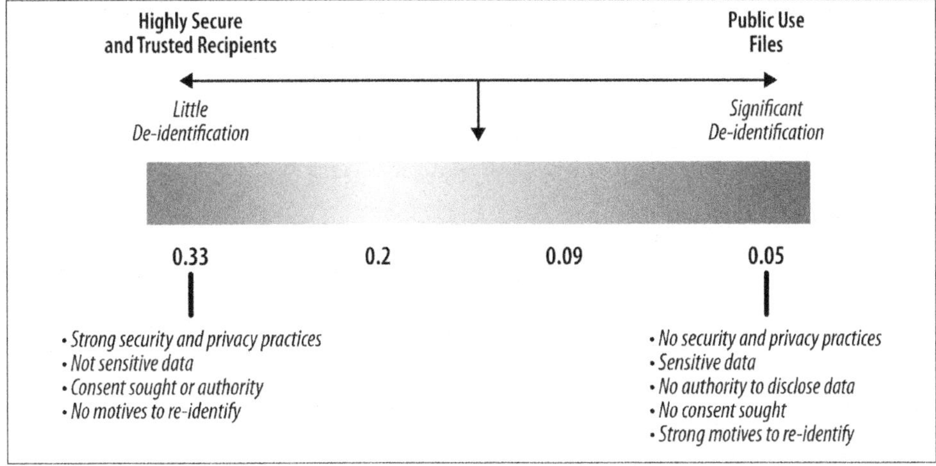

Figure 2-3. The different maximum risk thresholds that have been used in practice

To decide which threshold to use within this 0.09 to 0.05 range, we can look at the sensitivity of the data and the consent mechanism that was in place when the data was originally collected—this is the *invasion of privacy* dimension that needs to be evaluated.[1] For example, if the data is highly sensitive, we choose a lower threshold within that range. On the other hand, if the patients gave their explicit consent to releasing the data publicly while understanding the risks, we can set a higher threshold within that range.

What's Considered Sensitive Information?

All health data is sensitive. But some types of health information are considered especially sensitive because their disclosure is stigmatized or can be particularly harmful to the individual. What are these particularly harmful diagnoses? The National Committee on Vital Health Statistics has summarized what it believes can be considered "sensitive" information.[17]

Under federal law:

- Genetic information, including a disease or disorder in family members
- Psychotherapy notes recorded by a mental health professional providing care
- Substance abuse treatment records from almost any program

- Cash payments where the patient asks that it not be shared with a health insurance company

Under (many) state laws[18]):

- HIV information, or information on any sexually transmitted diseases
- Mental health information of any sort, including opinions formed or advice given regarding a patient's mental or emotional condition
- Information in the records of children and adolescents

For the sake of patient trust:

- Mental health information, beyond what's defined in state laws
- Sexuality and reproductive health information

When an entire record may be deemed sensitive:

- In cases of domestic violence or stalking
- When dealing with public figures and celebrities, or victims of violent crimes
- Records of adolescents, including childhood information

For data that's not publicly released, we have argued that the overall risk threshold should also be in the range of 0.1 to 0.05.[1] Let's take as an example a T1 attack. If the *Pr*(attempt) = 0.3, and the overall threshold was determined to be 0.1, then the threshold for *Pr*(re-id | attempt) = 0.1/0.3 = 0.33. This value is consistent with the precedents summarized in Figure 2-3. Choosing a threshold value in the 0.1 to 0.05 range is also a function of the *invasion of privacy* assessment.

By definition, average risk is equal to or lower than maximum risk. Arguably we should set thresholds for average risk that are equal to or lower than thresholds for maximum risk. On the other hand, attacks T1, T2, and T3 are on data sets that are not disclosed publicly, and, as we've discussed, they're very unlikely to result in a demonstration attack. So the thresholds used should really be higher than for T4. Based on a previous analysis, it's been recommended that the average risk thresholds vary between 0.1 and 0.05, depending on the results of an *invasion of privacy* score.[1] This balances the two competing requirements noted above. A summary is provided in Table 2-1.

Table 2-1. Attacks, risk metrics, and thresholds

Attack ID	Risk metric	Threshold range	Risk metric
T1	*Pr*(re-id, attempt)	0.1 to 0.05	Average risk
T2	*Pr*(re-id, acquaintance)	0.1 to 0.05	Average risk
T3	*Pr*(re-id, breach)	0.1 to 0.05	Average risk

Attack ID	Risk metric	Threshold range	Risk metric
T4	*Pr*(re-id)	0.09 to 0.05	Maximum risk

Meeting Thresholds

Once we've decided on a risk threshold, we then need a way to meet that threshold if the risk is found to be above it. We discussed what techniques to use to de-identify a data set in "Step 4: De-Identifying the Data" on page 28. At this point we're primarily interested in generalization and suppression. But how do you go about using these techniques to meet the risk threshold? First we need a couple of definitions:

Equivalence class
: All the records that have the same values on the quasi-identifiers. For example, all the records in a data set about 17-year-old males admitted on 2008/01/01[ii] are an equivalence class.

Equivalence class size
: The number of records in an equivalence class. Equivalence class sizes potentially change during de-identification. For example, there may be three records for 17-year-old males admitted on 2008/01/01. When the age is recoded to a five-year interval, then there may be eight records for males between 16 and 20 years old admitted on 2008/01/01.

k-anonymity
: The most common criterion to protect against re-identification. This states that the size of each equivalence class in the data set is at least *k*.[19] Many *k*-anonymity algorithms use generalization and suppression.

A simple example of de-identification using *k*-anonymity is illustrated in Figure 2-4. Here the objective was to achieve 3-anonymity through generalization and suppression. Each record pertains to a different patient, and there may be additional variables not shown because they're not quasi-identifiers. The de-identified data set in panel (b) has two equivalence classes (records 1, 2, 3, and 5, and records 7, 8, and 9), and three records were suppressed. We assume record suppression for simplicity, but in practice cell suppression could be used.

ii. We have adopted the ISO 8601 ordering of date elements, with yyyy/mm/dd, throughout the book.

(a)		
Admission Date	**Gender**	**Age**
2008/01/01	M	18
2008/01/01	M	17
2008/01/01	M	18
2008/01/01	M	13
2008/01/01	M	19
2008/01/01	F	18
2008/02/01	F	22
2008/02/01	F	23
2008/02/01	F	21
2008/01/01	M	22

(b)		
Admission Date	**Gender**	**Age**
2008/01/01	M	15-19
2008/01/01	M	15-19
2008/01/01	M	15-19
---	---	---
2008/01/01	M	15-19
---	---	---
2008/02/01	F	20-24
2008/02/01	F	20-24
2008/02/01	F	20-24
---	---	---

Figure 2-4. The original data set (a) de-identified into a 3-anonymous data set (b)

The basic attack that k-anonymity protects against assumes that the adversary has background information about a specific patient in the data set, and the adversary is trying to figure out which record belongs to that patient. The adversary might have the background information because he knows the patient personally (e.g., the patient is a neighbor, co-worker, or ex-spouse), or because the patient is famous and the information is public. But if there are at least k patients in the de-identified data set with the same values on their quasi-identifiers, the adversary has at most a $1/k$ chance of matching correctly to that patient. Now if we let k_i be the size of equivalence class i, then maximum risk is max(k_i) across all values of i in the data set, and average risk is average(k_i) across all values of i.

Risky Business

In many jurisdictions, demonstrating that a data set has a very small risk of re-identification is a legal or regulatory requirement. Our methodology provides a basis for meeting these requirements in a defensible, evidence-based way. But you need to follow all of the steps!

De-identification is no mean feat, and it requires a lot of forethought. The steps discussed in this chapter were formulated based on best practices that have evolved from a lot of academic and practical work. What we've done is break them down into digestible pieces so that you have a process to follow, leading to good data sharing practices of your own.

But the story doesn't end here, and there are plenty of details you can dig into.[1] We've only presented the highlights! We'll work through many examples throughout the book that shed light on the practical application of de-identification to real data sets, and we'll grow our repertoire of tools to deal with complex data sets and scenarios.

References

1. K. El Emam, *A Guide to the De-identification of Personal Health Information* (Boca Raton, FL: CRC Press/Auerbach, 2013).

2. U.S. Department of Health & Human Services, *Guidance Regarding Methods for De-identification of Protected Health Information in Accordance with the Health Insurance Portability and Accountability Act (HIPAA) Privacy Rule*, November 2012.

3. K. El Emam, A. Brown, and P. AbdelMalik, "Evaluating Predictors of Geographic Area Population Size Cut-Offs to Manage Re-Identification Risk," *Journal of the American Medical Informatics Association* 16:(2009): 256–266.

4. K. El Emam and P. Kosseim, "Privacy Interests in Prescription Data Part 2: Patient Privacy," *IEEE Security and Privacy* 7:7 (2009): 75–78.

5. K. El Emam, E. Jonker, L. Arbuckle, and B. Malin, "A Systematic Review of Re-identification Attacks on Health Data," *PLoS ONE* 6:12 (2001): e28071.

6. Y. Erlich, "Breaking Good: A Short Ethical Manifesto for the Privacy Researcher," (*http://bit.ly/breaking-good-report*) *Bill of Health*, 23 May 2013.

7. F. Dankar and K. El Emam, "Practicing Differential Privacy in Health Care: A Review," *Transactions on Data Privacy* 6:1 (2013): 35–67.

8. K.M. Stine, M.A. Scholl, P. Bowen, J. Hash, C.D. Smith, D. Steinberg, and L.A. Johnson, "An Introductory Resource Guide for Implementing the Health Insurance Portability and Accountability Act (HIPAA) Security Rule," NIST Special Publication 800-66 Revision 1, October 2008.

9. Symantec, *Symantec Global Internet Threat Report—Trends for July-December 07* (Symantec Enterprise Security, 2008).

10. B. Krebs, "Hackers Break into Virginia Health Professions Database, Demand Ransom," *Washington Post*, 4 May 2009.

11. J. Macfarlane, "Private medical records for sale: Harley Street clinic patients' files outsourced for computer input - and end up on black market," Mail Online, 18-Oct-2009.

12. S. Rubenstein, "Express Scripts Data Breach Leads to Extortion Attempt," *The Wall Street Journal*, 7 November 2008.

13. K. El Emam, F. Dankar, R. Issa, E. Jonker, D. Amyot, E. Cogo, J.-P. Corriveau, M. Walker, S. Chowdhury, R. Vaillancourt, T. Roffey, and J. Bottomley, "A Globally Optimal k-Anonymity Method for the De-identification of Health Data," *Journal of the American Medical Informatics Association* 16:5 (2009): 670–682.

14. J. Kim and J. Curry, "The Treatment of Missing Data in Multivariate Analysis," *Social Methods & Research* 6:(1977): 215–240.

15. R. Little and D. Rubin, *Statistical Analysis with Missing Data* (New York: John Wiley & Sons, 1987).

16. W. Vach and M. Blettner, "Biased Estimation of the Odds Ratio in Case-Control Studies Due to the Use of Ad Hoc Methods of Correcting for Missing Values for Confounding Variables," *American Journal of Epidemiology* 134:8 (1991): 895–907.

17. National Committee on Vital Health Statistics, letter to Kathleen Sebelius, Secretary to Department of Health and Human Services, 10 November 2010, "Re: Recommendations Regarding Sensitive Health Information."

18. American Health Lawyers Association,"State Healthcare Privacy Law Survey", 2013.

19. P. Samarati and L. Sweeney, "Protecting Privacy When Disclosing Information: *k*-Anonymity and Its Enforcement Through Generalisation and Suppression," Technical Report SRI-CSL-98-04 (Menlo Park, CA: SRI International, 1998).

CHAPTER 3

Cross-Sectional Data: Research Registries

One of the first real-life de-identification challenges we faced was releasing data from a maternal-child registry. It's common to create registries specifically to hold data that will be disclosed for secondary purposes. The Better Outcomes Registry & Network (BORN) of Ontario[1] integrates the data for all hospital and home births in the province, about 140,000 births per year. It was created for improving the provision of health care, and also for research. But without the ability to de-identify data sets, most research using this data would grind to a halt.

The data set from the BORN registry is cross-sectional, in that we cannot trace mothers over time. If a mother has a baby in 2009 and another in 2011, it's simply not possible to know that it was the same women. This kind of data is quite common in registries and surveys. We use the BORN data set a number of times throughout the book to illustrate various methods because it's a good baseline data set to work with and one that we know well.

Process Overview

We'll come back to BORN later. First we'll discuss the general process of getting de-identified data from a research registry.

Secondary Uses and Disclosures

Once the data is in the registry, outside researchers can make requests for access to data sets containing individual-level records. There's a process to approve these data requests, and it illustrates an important part of the de-identification process: health research studies need to be approved by Institutional Review Boards (IRBs) in the US or Research Ethics Boards (REBs) in Canada. We'll use REB for short since BORN is in Canada, but really our discussion applies equally to an IRB. REBs are often the only institutional gatekeepers providing oversight of research projects. Their primary mandate is to deal with the ethics of research studies, which means that they often deal with privacy issues. For example, the primary issues with many study protocols that involve the secondary analysis of data are related to privacy.

BORN for Research

What are some of the drivers that influence the rate of late preterm labor in Ontario? This was a question asked by researchers, and luckily for them BORN was able to produce a de-identified data set they could use to answer it! As a result of this work they were able to develop demographic tables and risk estimates for obstetrical factors and how they're associated with rates of late preterm birth (this work has been submitted for publication).

Does maternal exposure to air pollution influence the presence of obstetrical complications? BORN data was linked to pollution data to answer this question. Accurately linking the data required more information than would normally be allowed after de-identification, so instead it was done internally. The de-identified data set, with maternal and pollution data, was then provided to the research fellow working on this problem. The major finding was that preeclampsia is inversely proportional to moderate levels of carbon monoxide,[2] which is consistent with previous studies (although it's not yet clear why this relationship exists).

Does maternal H1N1 vaccination during pregnancy produce adverse infant and early childhood outcomes? Internal researchers at BORN linked maternal vaccination status from their own data to reported adverse childhood outcomes in the infants whose mothers were vaccinated (data provided by the Institute for Clinical Evaluative Sciences). This is ongoing research, but so far they've found that maternal vaccination during pregnancy is protective for the fetus and neonate.[3]

REBs shouldn't perform the de-identification of a data set, and arguably they aren't in a good position to determine whether a data set is de-identified or not. There are two main reasons for that:

- In practice, many REBs don't have privacy experts. It's simply not a requirement to have a privacy expert on the board. And even if there *is* a privacy expert, identifiability issues are a subdiscipline within privacy. General Counsel Jasmine, a privacy lawyer on the board, might be able to address questions around legislation and data use agreements, but she might not have the technical expertise to deal with questions about the identifiability of the data.
- The process of deciding whether a data set is identifiable and resolving re-identification risk concerns is iterative. Researcher Ronnie can easily agree to have dates of birth converted to ages, or to have admission and discharge dates converted to length of stay, if these are raised as presenting unacceptable re-identification risk.

But at the same time, Researcher Ronnie might not be happy with suppressing some records in the data set. This process of deciding on the trade-offs to convert an original data set to a de-identified data set that is still useful for the planned research requires negotiations with the researcher. The REB process and workflow is not well equipped for these types of iterative interactions, and if they are attempted they can be very slow and consequently frustrating.

An alternative approach that tends to work better in practice is for the re-identification risk assessment to be done prior to submitting a research protocol[i] to the REB. With this approach, Privacy Pippa, an expert on re-identification, works with Researcher Ronnie to decide how to manage the risk of re-identification through security controls and de-identification. This process is quite interactive and iterative. For this to work, an individual expert like Privacy Pippa must be assigned to the researcher by the organization holding the data, rather than the process being conducted by a committee that reviews data requests at, say, monthly meetings. Privacy Pippa could be assigned to work with multiple researchers at the same time, but it's always one expert per protocol. After Privacy Pippa and Researcher Ronnie have agreed on how to de-identify the data, a standard risk assessment report is produced and sent to the REB. We'll show you some simple examples of such a report at the end of this chapter.

The risk assessment report or certificate of de-identification the REB receives explains how the re-identification risk has been managed. This issue is then considered dealt with, and the board can move on to any other issues they have with the protocol. They're still accountable for the decision, but they essentially delegate the analysis to Privacy Pippa, who conducts the assessment and negotiations with Researcher Ronnie. Moving the re-identification risk assessment outside the board to the expert on de-identification ensures that the assessment is done thoroughly, that it's based on defensible evidence, and that the final outcome on this issue is satisfactory to the board as well as the researcher.

The REB also defines the acceptability criteria for the de-identification. For example, the board might say that the probability of re-identification must be below 0.2 for data that will be provided to researchers within the country, and 0.1 for researchers in other countries. Privacy Pippa would then use these as parameters for the assessment and negotiations with whatever researcher she's dealing with. The board might also stipulate other conditions, such as the requirement for Researcher Ronnie to sign a data sharing agreement. Privacy Pippa ensures that these conditions are met before the protocol is submitted to the board. This is the process that's in place with the BORN registry.

i. A research protocol outlines the methods and procedures that will be used to conduct the research.

Getting the Data

There's a process to getting health research data, summarized in Figure 3-1. The key players are Researcher Ronnie, a scientific review committee, a data access committee (DAC), the REB, and Database Administrator Darryl.

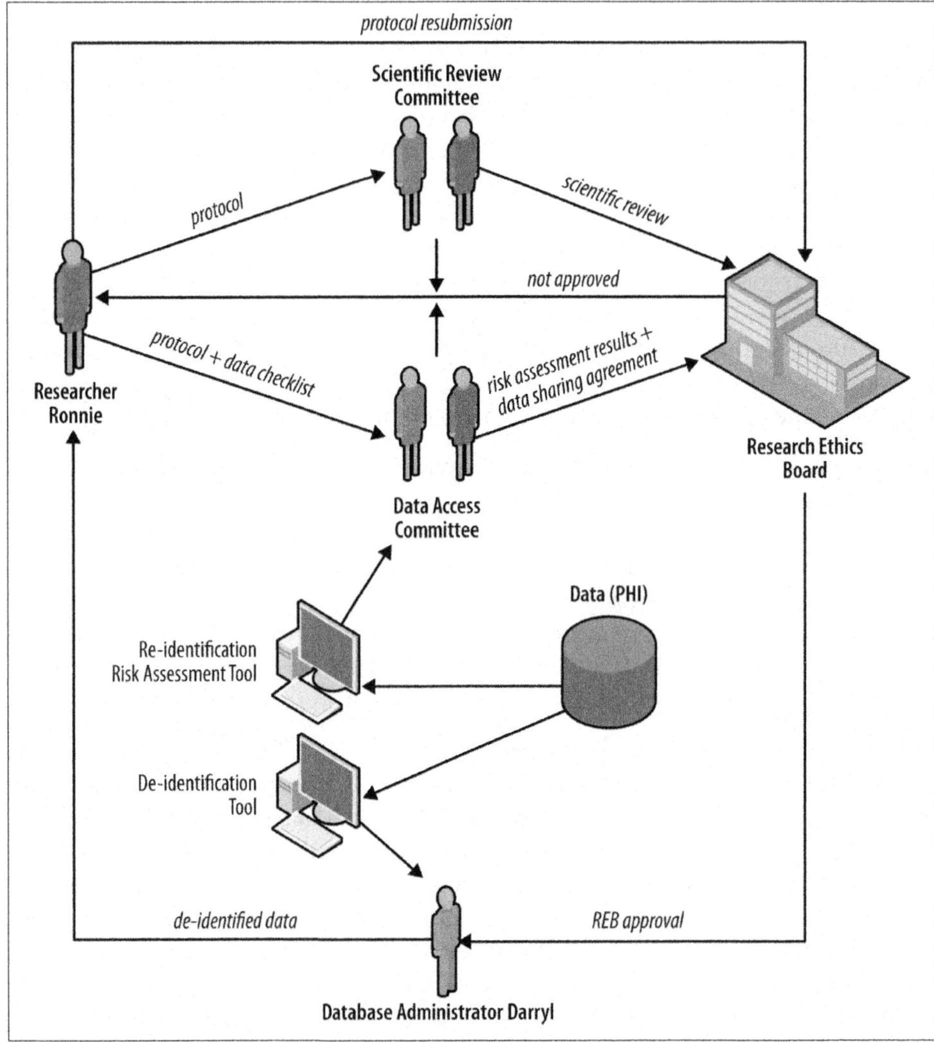

Figure 3-1. The process of getting health research data requires the involvement of a fair number of people

The scientific review committee might be a committee formed by a funding agency, or peers at a particular institution. The exact way that the scientific review is done isn't the topic of this book, but it's included here to illustrate a few key points. The DAC consists of de-identification and privacy experts who perform a re-identification risk assessment on the protocol.

The DAC needs to have access to tools that can perform a re-identification risk assessment. These tools also need to be able to analyze the original data being requested in order to perform that risk assessment. Database Administrator Darryl is responsible for holding on securely to data with protected health information (PHI) and has an appropriate de-identification tool in place to de-identify the data.

Creating a Functional DAC

In setting up the DAC, there are a number of critical success factors to consider:

Expertise
: The HIPAA Privacy Rule (*http://1.usa.gov/privacy-impacts*) defines a de-identification expert as "a person with appropriate knowledge of and experience with generally accepted statistical and scientific principles and methods for rendering information not individually identifiable." Only recently have applied courses started coming out that can help individuals develop the necessary expertise—these should start having an impact on the available pool of experts soon. Having a well-defined methodology to follow, like we describe in this book, should provide concrete guidance on the steps to consider and the issues to address specifically for health data.

Duration
: One of the common complaints about the use of de-identification experts is that the process takes a long time. If we add another layer into the data release process, in the form of the DAC, will this further slow access to data? Automation could help speed up some of the iterative analysis that needs to be done, and it also reduces the amount of detailed knowledge that a DAC member needs to acquire. A key is to also have dedicated resources in the DAC.

Performance measurement
: Measuring the performance of the DAC in general is quite important. The dedicated DAC resources can then be evaluated on a well-defined set of metrics, and this creates an incentive to optimize on these metrics. Useful metrics would include turnaround time and researcher satisfaction (as measured through surveys).

Formulating the Protocol

Researcher Ronnie submits the research protocol to the scientific review committee and the DAC. In practice there might be some iteration between the scientific review process and the DAC process.

The DAC performs a re-identification risk assessment and decides how to adequately de-identify the data set requested by Researcher Ronnie. This process might result in changing the precision of the data that's requested. For example, the original protocol might request admission and discharge dates, but the risk assessment might recommend replacing that with length of stay in days. Such changes in the data might require changes in the protocol as well.

If the protocol changes, the scientific review might have to be revisited. Also, during the scientific review, methodological or theoretical issues might be raised that could affect the requested data elements. If the requested data elements change, the re-identification risk assessment might have to be revisited. Therefore, at least conceptually, there's potentially some interaction and possibly iteration between the scientific review process and the re-identification risk assessment process performed by the DAC.

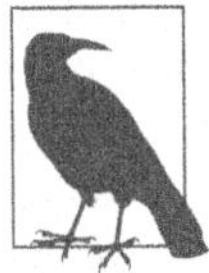

In practice, the interaction between scientific review and data access review isn't often possible because of the way peer review is structured (e.g., with the research funding agencies). Since there's not likely to be any interaction or iteration between scientific review and data access review, we can save time by doing these activities in parallel, or sequence them and hope for the best!

If either the scientific review committee or the DAC doesn't approve the protocol, it goes back to Researcher Ronnie for a revision. If the scientific review committee approves the protocol, it provides some kind of approval documentation, such as a letter.

Negotiating with the Data Access Committee

Researcher Ronnie provides the DAC with the protocol as well as a variable checklist. This checklist is quite important because it clarifies the exact fields that are requested. It also highlights to Researcher Ronnie which fields in the requested database are quasi-identifiers and might therefore undergo some kind of generalization and suppression.

The checklist allows Researcher Ronnie to indicate the level of data granularity that he'll accept. For example, he might be willing to get the year of birth instead of the full date of birth. If this is explicitly specified up front in the checklist, it will most likely reduce significantly the number of iterations between Researcher Ronnie and the DAC. The checklist should also contain information about the importance of the quasi-identifiers —an important quasi-identifier should be minimally impacted by the de-identification. The more trade-offs that Researcher Ronnie is willing to make up front, the less time the re-identification risk analysis will require.

The DAC determines how to appropriately de-identify the data given the risks, and negotiates the chosen process with Researcher Ronnie. This negotiation could take a number of iterations, but these iterations should be relatively quick because a single individual from the DAC is assigned to negotiate with the researcher. The point is not to create another layer of bureaucracy, but to negotiate trade-offs. The output from this process consists of two things:

Risk assessment results
: This consists of a report indicating the de-identification that will be applied as well as the residual risk in the data set that will be disclosed. We'll provide an example in "Risk Assessment" on page 53.

Data sharing agreement
: Because the amount of de-identification would normally be contingent on the security and privacy practices that Researcher Ronnie has in place, he must commit to implementing these practices in a data sharing agreement. This agreement isn't always needed. For example, if Researcher Ronnie is an employee of a hospital and the data comes from the hospital, then he will be bound by an employment contract that should cover the handling of sensitive patient data. However, if Researcher Ronnie is external to the hospital or at a university, then a data sharing agreement would most certainly be recommended. A different data sharing agreement would be needed for every project because the specific terms may vary depending on the data required.

Once it gets these two items, the REB will have sufficient evidence that the residual risk of re-identification is acceptably low and will know the terms of the data sharing agreement that Researcher Ronnie will be signing for this particular data release. There's evidence that many Canadian REBs will waive the requirement to obtain patient consent if they're convinced that the requested data set is de-identified. And now the REB can perform a regular ethics review knowing that the privacy issues have been addressed.

If the REB approves the protocol, this information is conveyed to Database Administrator Darryl, who then creates a data set according to the risk assessment report. Database Administrator Darryl then provides the data to Researcher Ronnie in some secure format.

If the REB doesn't approve the protocol for reasons not related to re-identification risk, Researcher Ronnie has to resubmit the protocol at some later point with the changes required by the REB. If the protocol isn't approved because of an issue related to re-identification risk, Researcher Ronnie has to go through the process again with the DAC to perform another risk assessment.

BORN Ontario

Now back to our case study. BORN is a prescribed registry under Ontario's health privacy legislation, and is allowed to use and disclose the data collected. But it's obligated to protect the personal health information of mothers and their babies. Now, that doesn't mean it has to lock it down—it wants the data to be used to improve the maternal-child health care system. But this legislation does mean that there must be safeguards in place, which we'll get to.

The data is collected through a number of mechanisms, including manual data entry and automated extraction and uploads from health record systems. The registry includes information about the infants' and mothers' health. Several sources contribute to the data collected by BORN:

- Prenatal screening labs
- Hospitals (labor, birth, and early newborn care information including NICU admissions)
- Midwifery groups (labor, birth, and early newborn care information)
- Specialized antenatal clinics (information about congenital anomalies)
- Newborn screening labs
- Prenatal screening and newborn screening follow-up clinics
- Fertility clinics

BORN Data Set

Researchers will request all kinds of data sets from BORN to answer interesting questions relating to mothers and their children. The sidebar "BORN for Research" on page 46 gives a few examples, but let's just take one simple example to demonstrate the process we've been describing.

Researcher Ronnie at an Ontario university made a request for the clinical records in the registry. The registry doesn't collect any direct identifiers, such as names or social insurance numbers, so a researcher can only request indirect identifiers and clinical variables. There are a lot of variables in the registry, so we'll focus on the fields that were requested.

No specific cohort was requested by Researcher Ronnie, so all records in the registry were included, from 2005–2011. At the time of analysis the registry had 919,710 records. The fields requested are summarized in Table 3-1. These are the quasi-identifiers, because fields that are direct identifiers can't be released at all. Researcher Ronnie didn't request highly sensitive data, such as data on congenital anomalies or maternal health problems, which plays a role in our selection of a risk threshold.

Table 3-1. Quasi-identifiers requested by Researcher Ronnie

Field	Description
BSex	Baby's sex
MDOB	Maternal date of birth
BDOB	Baby's date of birth
MPC	Maternal postal code

We can't generalize the sex variable, but a *generalization hierarchy* was defined for each of the other three variables, shown in Table 3-2. A generalization hierarchy is a list of changes that the organization could potentially apply to the data, arranged from the most specific (and most risky) representation to a less specific (and safer) representation.

Table 3-2. Generalization hierarchy for the quasi-identifiers

Field	Generalization hierarchy
MDOB	dd/mm/year → week/year → mm/year → quarter/year → year → 5-year interval → 10-year interval
BDOB	dd/mm/year → week/year → mm/year → quarter/year → year → 5-year interval → 10-year interval
MPC	Cropping the last *x* character(s), where *x* is 1 → 2 → 3 → 4 → 5

Risk Assessment

Based on a detailed risk assessment, as described in "Step 2: Setting the Threshold" on page 25, we determined that an average risk threshold of 0.1 would be appropriate for Researcher Ronnie and the data he requested. Had he requested highly sensitive variables, such as data on congenital anomalies or maternal health problems, the risk threshold would have been set to 0.05.

Threat Modeling

Now we examine the three plausible attacks for a known data recipient that were discussed in "Step 3: Examining Plausible Attacks" on page 26:

1. For a deliberate attempt at re-identification, we need to set the value for the probability of attempt, *Pr*(attempt), based on expert opinion. In this case the researcher was at an academic institution with a data agreement in place, in the same country, and with no obvious reason to want to re-identify records in the registry (low motives and capacity). That being said, Researcher Ronnie didn't have much in the way of security and privacy practices, just the bare minimum (low mitigating controls). So although the data wasn't sensitive, the detailed risk assessment concluded that an appropriate estimate would be *Pr*(attempt) = 0.4.
2. Evaluating an inadvertent attempt at re-identification requires an estimate of the probability that a researcher will have an acquaintance in the data set, *Pr*(acquaint-

ance). A first estimate would simply be the probability of knowing a woman that has had a baby in any one year between 2005–2011 (assuming that Researcher Ronnie at least knows the year of birth). The worst-case estimate would be based on the year 2008, in which there were 119,785 births out of 4,478,500 women between the ages of 14 and 60. That's a prevalence of 0.027, which results in $Pr(\text{acquaintance}) = 1-(1-0.027)^{150/2} = 0.87$. In this case we divided the estimated number of friends, 150, in half because we were only considering women (male pregnancies would most certainly be outliers!).

3. For a data breach we already have $Pr(\text{breach}) = 0.27$, based on historical data.

Our basic measure of risk boils down to $Pr(\text{re-id}, \text{T}) = Pr(\text{T}) \times Pr(\text{re-id} \mid \text{T})$, where the factor $Pr(\text{T})$ is one of the previously mentioned probabilities. The higher the value of $Pr(\text{T})$, the more de-identification we need to perform on the data set. So in this case we were most concerned with an inadvertent attempt at re-identification, with $Pr(\text{re-id}, \text{acquaintance}) = 0.87 \times Pr(\text{re-id} \mid \text{acquaintance}) \leq 0.1$, where the last factor was determined directly from the data set. We therefore have $Pr(\text{re-id} \mid \text{acquaintance}) \leq 0.115$.

Results

With a risk threshold in hand, and a generalization hierarchy to work with, we produced a de-identified data set with a minimized amount of cell suppression.[4] Our first attempt resulted in a data set with MDOB in year, BDOB in week/year, and MPCs of one character, leading to the missingness and entropy shown in Table 3-3. These are the same measures we first saw in "Information Loss Metrics" on page 35.

Table 3-3. First attempt at de-identification

	Cell missingness	Record missingness	Entropy
Before	0.02%	0.08%	
After	0.75%	0.79%	58.26%

Researcher Ronnie explained that geography was more important than we had originally thought, and suggested that the first three digits of postal codes would provide the geographic resolution he needed. He also clarified that the mother's date of birth didn't need to be overly precise. So we made it possible to increase the precision of the postal code, without increasing risk, by decreasing the precision of other measures. Our second attempt resulted in a data set with MDOB in 10-year intervals, BDOB in quarter/year, and MPCs of three characters, leading to the missingness and entropy values in Table 3-4.

Table 3-4. Second attempt at de-identification

	Cell missingness	Record missingness	Entropy
Before	0.02%	0.08%	
After	0.02%	0.08%	64.24%

Entropy increased here because of the large change in the level of generalization of the mother's date of birth. But given that no noticeable suppression was applied to the data, Researcher Ronnie asked that we try to increase the precision of the baby's date of birth. Our third attempt resulted in a data set with MDOB in 10-year intervals, BDOB in month/year, and MPCs of three characters, leading to the missingness and entropy values in Table 3-5.

Table 3-5. Third attempt at de-identification

	Cell missingness	Record missingness	Entropy
Before	0.02%	0.08%	
After	26.7%	26.7%	59.59%

Given the massive increase in missingness, Researcher Ronnie requested the second attempt at producing a de-identified data set, with MDOB in 10-year intervals, BDOB in quarter/year, and MPCs of three characters, leading to the missingness and entropy values in Table 3-4.

Year on Year: Reusing Risk Analyses

Let's say Researcher Ronnie had only asked for a data set for one particular year, say 2005. The next year he decides to run a follow-up study and asks for the same data, but for 2006 (he no longer has the 2005 data, because it was deleted as part of the data retention rules). Can we use the same de-identification scheme that we used for the 2005 data, with the same generalizations, or do we need to do a new risk assessment on the 2006 data? If the de-identification specifications are different, it will be difficult to pool statistical results.

This question comes up a lot, so we decided to test it using BORN data sets from the years 2005–2010. The initial size and missingness for the data sets for each year are shown in Table 3-6. We applied our de-identification algorithm to the 2005 data set first, using the same risk threshold of 0.115 as before. With BSex unchanged, the result was MDOB in year, BDOB in week/year, and MPCs of three characters.

Table 3-6. Summary of data sets over six years

Year	No. of records	Cell missingness	Record missingness
2005	114,352	0.02%	0.07%
2006	119,785	0.01%	0.06%

Year	No. of records	Cell missingness	Record missingness
2007	129,540	0.02%	0.06%
2008	137,122	0.02%	0.07%
2009	138,926	0.01%	0.05%
2010	137,351	0.03%	0.14%

We then applied exactly the same generalizations to each of the subsequent years, from 2006–2010. Suppression was applied until the average risk was below our threshold of 0.115. The results for the remaining years are shown in Table 3-7, and as you can see they're quite stable across years. This means that, for this data set, there's no need to re-evaluate the risk of re-identification for subsequent years. There are a couple of advantages to this result:

- We can do re-identification risk assessments on subsets, knowing that we would get the same results if we ran the analysis on the full data set. This can reduce computation time.
- It allows BORN to have a data sharing agreement in place and provide data sets to researchers on an annual basis using the same specification without having to re-do all of the analysis again.

Table 3-7. De-identification over six years, using the same generalizations

Year	Cell missingness	Record missingness	Entropy
2005	3.41%	3.42%	61.04%
2006	2.54%	2.54%	61.27%
2007	1.64%	1.65%	61.28%
2008	1.24%	1.26%	61.26%
2009	1.15%	1.16%	61.25%
2010	1.42%	1.47%	61.23%

That being said, the BORN data pertains to very stable populations—newborns and their mothers. There haven't been dramatic changes in the number or characteristics of births in Ontario from 2005–2010. The stability of the data contributes to the stability of de-identification. If we had changed the group of quasi-identifiers used from one year to the next, the results would not hold.

Final Thoughts

There are a lot of people overseeing access to data in the health care system, and that's a good thing. But luckily, there's usually a system in place to release the data for secondary purposes, especially research. Evidence-based health care requires data, and patients want their privacy. Together they have driven the need for a process of access with oversight.

Sometimes researchers expect that de-identification will not give them useful data. However, if done properly this is not going to be the case. The key point to remember, at least with regard to de-identification, is that the researcher needs to know the process and be prepared to negotiate with respect to the controls that need to be put in place, the available data elements, and the trade-offs needed to ensure the utility of information given the intended analysis.

After negotiating with a DAC, the de-identification risk assessment results need to be provided to a research ethics or institutional review board; this is a key reason for documenting the process of de-identification.

We get asked a lot about stability of de-identification, and with the BORN data we were able to show that, at least with a stable population, it seems to hold its own. But it's a good idea to revisit a de-identification scheme every 18 to 24 months to ensure that there haven't been any material changes to the data set and the processes that generate it. And to be clear, the de-identification scheme should be revisited if any quasi-identifiers are added or changed—that would be considered a material change.

References

1. The Better Outcomes Registry & Network (BORN) of Ontario (*http://www.bornontario.ca*)

2. D. Zhai, Y. Guo, G. Smith, D. Krewski, M. Walker, and S.W. Wen, "Maternal Exposure to Moderate Ambient Carbon Monoxide Is Associated with Decreased Risk of Preeclampsia," *American Journal of Obstetrics & Gynecology*, 207:1 (2012): 57.e1–9.

3. B. Deshayne, A.E. Sprague, N. Liu, A.S. Yasseen, S.W. Wen, G. Smith, and M.C. Walker, "H1N1 Influenza Vaccination During Pregnancy and Fetal and Neonatal Outcomes," *American Journal of Public Health* 102:(2012): e33-e40.

4. K. El Emam, F. Dankar, R. Issa, E. Jonker, D. Amyot, E. Cogo, J.-P. Corriveau, M. Walker, S. Chowdhury, R. Vaillancourt, T. Roffey, and J. Bottomley, "A Globally Optimal *k*-Anonymity Method for the De-identification of Health Data," *Journal of the American Medical Informatics Association* 16:5 (2009): 670–682.

CHAPTER 4

Longitudinal Discharge Abstract Data: State Inpatient Databases

After patients are discharged from a hospital—in some cases months after—their medical information is organized and cleaned up to accurately reflect their stay in the hospital. The resulting document is known as a *discharge abstract*. A State Inpatient Database (SID) is a collection of all Discharge Abstract Data (DAD) for a state, and it's a powerful tool for research and analysis to inform public policy.[1]

The SID databases for many states are made available for research and other purposes. But there have been concerns raised about how well they've been de-identified when shared,[2] and some have been successfully attacked.[3] We'll provide some analysis to inform de-identification practices for this kind of data, and we'll look at methods that can be used to create a public use SID.

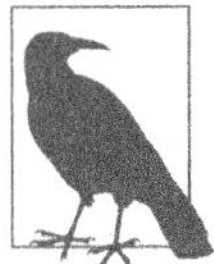

In addition to quasi-identifiers, a data set can contain sensitive information such as drugs dispensed or diagnoses. This information could be used to infer things like mental health status or disabilities. We don't consider that kind of sensitive information in the analysis here, for ease of presentation, but just assume that it exists in the data sets we refer to. Re-identifying patients therefore implies potentially learning about sensitive information that patients might not want others to know about.

While we'll present de-identification algorithms here in the context of longitudinal data, any multilevel data set can be de-identified using these methods as well. A birth registry with maternal information at the first level could, for example, be combined with information about each baby at the second level, or data about cancer patients at the top level could be combined with data about their family members who've had cancer at the second level.

Longitudinal Data

Over a period of time, patients can make multiple hospital or clinic visits, and linking a patient's records throughout is what makes the data *longitudinal*. Data sets of this type need to be de-identified differently from cross-sectional data. If you try to de-identify a longitudinal data set using methods developed for cross-sectional data, you'll either do too little to protect the patients properly, or you'll do too much and distort the data to the point where it becomes useless.

We can understand this principle by looking at the example of longitudinal data in Figure 4-1. There are six patients with basic demographics in panel (a), and their visit information in panel (b). ZIP codes were collected at each visit in case patients moved. The patients with IDs 10 and 11 had three visits each in 2009, whereas patient 12 had only two visits: one in 2008 and one in 2009. The patient ID (PID) is used to identify the visits that belong to a patient—without it we'd lose the longitudinal nature of the data set, and lose the chance to do any analysis benefitting from a survey of multiple visits by a patient. In addition, at least for this data set, we wouldn't be able to link to patient demographics.

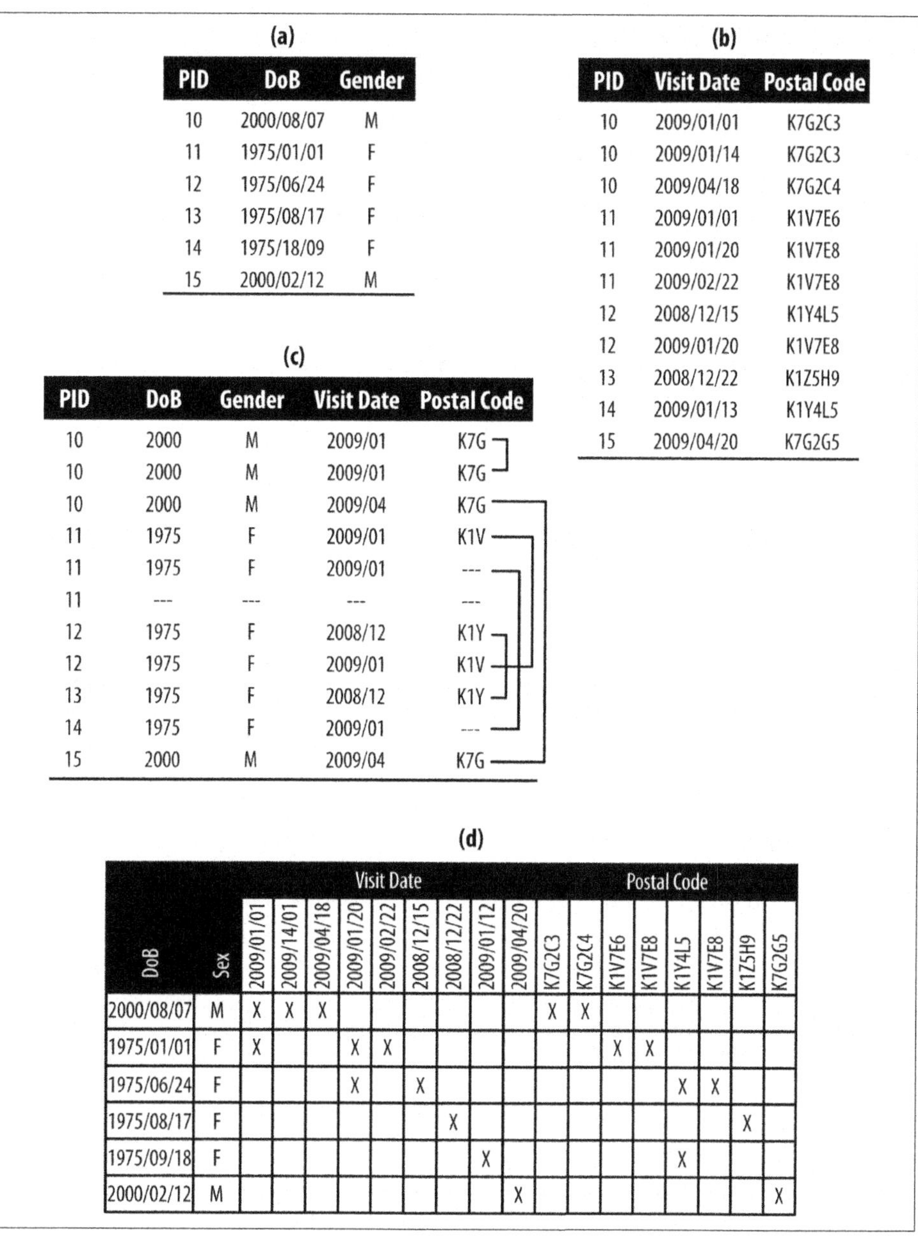

(a)

PID	DoB	Gender
10	2000/08/07	M
11	1975/01/01	F
12	1975/06/24	F
13	1975/08/17	F
14	1975/18/09	F
15	2000/02/12	M

(b)

PID	Visit Date	Postal Code
10	2009/01/01	K7G2C3
10	2009/01/14	K7G2C3
10	2009/04/18	K7G2C4
11	2009/01/01	K1V7E6
11	2009/01/20	K1V7E8
11	2009/02/22	K1V7E8
12	2008/12/15	K1Y4L5
12	2009/01/20	K1V7E8
13	2008/12/22	K1Z5H9
14	2009/01/13	K1Y4L5
15	2009/04/20	K7G2G5

(c)

PID	DoB	Gender	Visit Date	Postal Code
10	2000	M	2009/01	K7G
10	2000	M	2009/01	K7G
10	2000	M	2009/04	K7G
11	1975	F	2009/01	K1V
11	1975	F	2009/01	---
11	---	---	---	---
12	1975	F	2008/12	K1Y
12	1975	F	2009/01	K1V
13	1975	F	2008/12	K1Y
14	1975	F	2009/01	---
15	2000	M	2009/04	K7G

(d)

		Visit Date									Postal Code							
DoB	Sex	2009/01/01	2009/14/01	2009/04/18	2009/01/20	2009/02/22	2008/12/15	2008/12/22	2009/01/12	2009/04/20	K7G2C3	K7G2C4	K1V7E6	K1V7E8	K1Y4L5	K1V7E8	K1Z5H9	K7G2G5
2000/08/07	M	X	X	X							X	X						
1975/01/01	F	X			X	X							X	X				
1975/06/24	F				X		X								X	X		
1975/08/17	F							X									X	
1975/09/18	F								X						X			
2000/02/12	M									X								X

Figure 4-1. Demographics (a) and visits (b), joined and 2-anonymized (c), with a binary view (d) for good measure

Don't Treat It Like Cross-Sectional Data

k-anonymization techniques using generalization and suppression for de-identifying cross-sectional data won't work as intended on longitudinal data. To see why, let's try some techniques from the previous chapter on our example longitudinal data and see the problems that arise:

Suppression in single records
: One way to represent the longitudinal data in Figure 4-1 is to join the two tables in panels (a) and (b) and have a single data set of patient visits. Each patient can appear multiple times in the joined data set. Panel (c) in Figure 4-1 shows what this de-identified data set with 2-anonymity would look like. The postal code for patient number 11 was suppressed in her second visit, and all quasi-identifiers for her third visit were suppressed. But k-anonymity treats each record as an independent observation, ignoring the PID entirely. An adversary could see that the first and second visit are in the same month, and guess that the first three digits of the patient's postal code won't have changed. The postal code was suppressed to achieve 2-anonymity, but it didn't actually work as intended.

Homogeneous equivalence classes
: The probability of re-identifying a patient is not necessarily as low as intended when applying current k-anonymity algorithms to longitudinal data. Under k-anonymity, the first two records in panel (c) of Figure 4-1 form an equivalence class. But the records belong to the same patient, so the probability of re-identifying the patient is 1 despite having $k = 2$.

Detailed background knowledge
: Let's say that an adversary wants to re-identify Alice in the data. The adversary has collected some information about her and knows that she's made at least a couple of visits to the hospital. In our example data, two female patients have made at least two visits to the hospital. But the adversary knows that Alice's visits were in "2008/11 and 2009/01." That makes her PID 12. Because k-anonymity treats a data set as cross-sectional, patterns that span multiple records (i.e., longitudinal patterns) are not protected.

Another way to represent such longitudinal data is by creating a variable for each quasi-identifier. This is referred to as *binary* or *transactional data*. We show this in panel (d) of Figure 4-1. This kind of representation has been used to evaluate re-identification risk for patient location trails,[4,5] and to de-identify transactions.[6,7] The variables for a location trail could be a set of hospitals that were visited; the variables for transactions could be a set of drugs that were purchased.

The k-anonymity techniques used for this kind of data will ensure that there are no equivalence classes smaller than k. But as you can probably imagine, this setup can result in a large number of variables, and a high-dimensional data set. And that, in turn, will lead to heavy information loss.[8] In other words, most of the cells in the table will be suppressed, and the resulting de-identified data set will be nearly useless.

De-Identifying Under Complete Knowledge

At this point it's pretty clear that we need a different way to suppress cells and manage risk in longitudinal data—treating longitudinal data as cross-sectional just won't cut it. Treating longitudinal data responsibly, which involves accounting for the multiple records for a single patient, is necessary to ensure proper de-identification.

Let's start by representing the longitudinal data in a new way, as a two-level tree. The first level contains the patient's demographics, which don't change across visits; the second level contains the patient's visits. PID 10, for instance, has three visits, shown as a two-level tree in Figure 4-2.

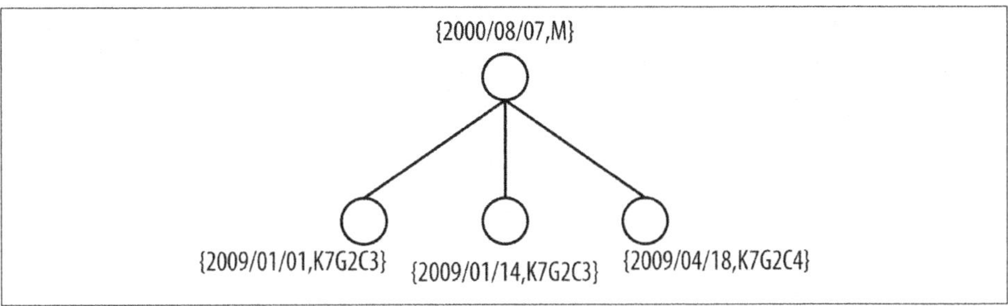

Figure 4-2. PID 10 pretending to be a tree: demographics (level 1), visits (level 2)

Under the assumption of complete knowledge, we assume that an adversary knows about all of the visits for a specific patient. For PID 10 (Figure 4-2) this means the adversary knows the patient's date of birth (DOB), gender, the exact dates when he visited the hospital, and where he lived at the time (i.e., his postal code)... stalker! In short, complete knowledge is a worst-case assumption because the adversary knows everything there is to know from the quasi-identifiers. This is a lot of information, but it's a starting point for developing new ways to assess and manage the risk from longitudinal data. We'll look at ways of relaxing these assumptions later.

Here's the problem: we don't know which patient will be targeted. So there's no choice but to protect all patients against an adversary with complete knowledge. This means that we have to protect against an adversary with complete knowledge for all patients with one visit, for all patients with two visits, for all patients with three visits... for all patients with any number of visits!

But we do have one saving grace: *exact* versus *approximate* complete knowledge. Exact complete knowledge is what we've described already. Approximate complete knowledge gives us some leeway because the quasi-identifier values are treated as independent sets.

For PID 10, the adversary would know the visit dates {2009/01/01, 2009/01/14, 2009/04/18} and postal codes {K7G2C3, K7G2C3, K7G2C4}, but not which postal codes go with which visit dates. "Approximate" here means that the adversary has all the pieces of information, but doesn't know how they are connected to each other in visits.

This might seem extreme. How can an adversary that knows dates of visits not know where the target lives? But keep in mind that this is already a *lot* of information to know about someone. Maybe the adversary knows that the target has moved around a few times, perhaps to a new neighborhood and then back because they preferred the old neighborhood. Maybe the adversary worked at a café near the clinic where the target was seeking treatment, and they've chatted. So she knows a lot, but has forgotten how to piece all that information together. The point, rather, is to relax the very strict and conservative assumptions of exact complete knowledge. But if we don't like an assumption, and we want to connect dates to postal codes even for approximate complete knowledge, we most certainly can.

Connected Variables

There are times when you need to connect variables during de-identification so that they're treated more or less the same. We consider two basic types of connections:

QI to QI
: Sometimes quasi-identifiers are so similar that their de-identification needs to be connected so that both are generalized and suppressed in the same way. Date of delivery and maternal date of discharge are connected because they are strongly correlated—discharge is usually two days after delivery. This means that if you know one you can accurately predict the other. You wouldn't want one of these dates to be given in weeks and the other in months, which could happen if the two variables weren't explicitly connected. Another example would be the date of a clinic visit and the date in the log file from an electronic medical record. These two dates will likely be exactly the same because entries in the medical record will happen on the date of the visit. Typically you would connect QIs that are of the same type so that generalizations will be linked and done in the same way.

QI to non-QI
: Many quasi-identifiers are coded in some way (e.g., *1* for natural childbirth, *2* for Cesarean), and include a description field to explain what the codes mean without having to look elsewhere. Suppressing the coded value but not the accompanying description would be no different than not doing any suppression at all! Clearly these two fields need to be connected so that suppression is done on both. We see this type of connectedness often in data, with diagnosis, procedure, and drug codes, not to mention any site-specific custom codes. Without a description field these codes become almost meaningless because there are literally thousands of them.

In general, approximate complete knowledge is probably more practical, because exact complete knowledge is so very strong an assumption. Both could be tried as a form of sensitivity analysis to determine their impact on the data. Which one you assume may ultimately depend on how conservative you want to be while preserving data quality. Assuming even approximate complete knowledge may actually be too strong an assumption if there are a significant number of visits, but that's something we'll discuss in a later chapter. First let's look at these concepts in more detail.

Approximate Complete Knowledge

Let's consider a new data set, given in panel (a) of Figure 4-3. We'll group patients by the number of visits they had, and flatten the data so each patient is in one row. We've done this in panel (b), and performed some generalization to get us close to 2-anonymity. Structuring the data as a series of flat files, based on the number of visits, allows us to use *k*-anonymity. After all, we don't want to throw out the baby with the bathwater!

Our generalization in panel (b) got us close to 2-anonymity:

One-visit patients
: The first and third patients make an equivalence class of size 2, and the second patient has to be flagged for suppression because she is in an equivalence class of size 1.

Three-visit patients
: The visits and postal codes are ordered. The two patients match exactly, creating an equivalence class of size 2.

For approximate complete knowledge, we assume that the adversary doesn't know which combinations of visit date and postal code go together. An adversary might know, for instance, that the first patient was born in 1975, had two visits in 2009/01 and a visit in 2009/04, and lived at K7D for one visit and at K7G for two visits.

(a)

PID	DoB	Gender
100	1975/08/07	M
101	1975/01/01	M
102	1975/06/24	F
103	1975/08/17	F
104	1975/09/18	F

PID	VID	Visit Date	Postal Code
100	1	2009/01/01	K7G2C3
100	2	2009/01/14	K7G2G5
100	3	2009/04/18	K7D2C3
101	4	2009/01/01	K7D2C4
101	5	2009/04/18	K7G2C3
101	6	2009/01/14	K7G2G3
102	7	2009/01/20	K1V7E8
103	8	2008/12/22	K1Z5H9
104	9	2009/01/13	K1V4L5

(b)

DoB	Gender	Visit Date 1	Postal Code 1
1975	F	2009/01	K1V
1975	F	2008/12	K1Z
1975	F	2009/01	K1V

1 Visit Patients

DoB	Gender	Visit Date 1	Visit Date 2	Visit Date 3	Postal Code 1	Postal Code 2	Postal Code 3
1975	M	2009/01	2009/01	2009/04	K7D	K7G	K7G
1975	M	2009/01	2009/01	2009/04	K7D	K7G	K7G

3 Visit Patients

(c)

DoB	Gender	Visit 1
1975	F	(2009/01, K1V)
1975	F	(2008/12, K1Z)
1975	F	(2009/01, K1V)

1 Visit Patients

DoB	Gender	Visit 1	Visit 2	Visit 3
1975	M	(2009/01, K7G)	(2009/01, K7G)	(2009/04, K7D)
1975	M	(2009/01, K7D)	(2009/01, K7G)	(2009/04, K7G)

3 Visit Patients

Figure 4-3. The original data (a) under approximate complete knowledge (b) and exact complete knowledge (c)

Exact Complete Knowledge

If we assume exact complete knowledge, we still want to group patients by the number of visits they had and flatten the data so each patient is in one row. But this time, in panel

(c) of Figure 4-3, we keep the visit dates and postal codes together as pairs. So, we're keeping the visit data together before we apply *k*-anonymity.

Our generalization in panel (c) is the same as before, and gets us close to 2-anonymity:

One-visit patients
: The results are the same as before—the second patient has to be flagged for suppression.

Three-visit patients
: This time patients don't match on the first and third visits, because of the postal codes. Both patients therefore have to be flagged for suppression.

Exact complete knowledge is a stricter assumption, leading to more de-identification. In our example, two more patients had to be flagged for suppression than with approximate complete knowledge.

If the longitudinal patterns were more similar, or homogeneous, there would be less difference between exact and approximate knowledge. For example, if patients didn't move, then their postal codes wouldn't change, and there would be much less to de-identify. On the flip side, if the longitudinal patterns were less similar, or heterogeneous, there would be a greater difference between exact and approximate knowledge.

Implementation

The implementation of the *k*-anonymity checks described in the previous sections would not require the creation of multiple tables in practice (i.e., one table for each number of visits). For approximate complete knowledge, each of the values would be represented by its hash value (a hash is a really fast way to identify and filter duplicate information). This would speed up the comparisons of values to compute equivalence classes, and where the values need to be ordered for comparison (for patients with more than one visit), the ordering is performed on the hash values as well. The actual ordering chosen does not actually matter as long as the ordering is performed consistently for all patient records.

The level 2 values for the three-visit patients in panel (b) of Figure 4-3 are ordered by year for dates and alphabetically for postal codes. When hashed, the ordering would be on the hashed values and this would give the same result. An alternative would be to use a commutative hash function, in which case the order would not matter.

Generalization Under Complete Knowledge

The demographics at level 1, DOB and gender, are generalized in the same way as for cross-sectional data, using a generalization hierarchy (like we saw in "BORN Data Set" on page 52). The visit information at level 2, date, and postal code, is generalized in the same way for all visits in the data set. If we generalize the visit date to the year of visit, all of the visit dates for all patients would be generalized to year.

The State Inpatient Database (SID) of California

State Inpatient Databases (SIDs) were developed as part of the Healthcare Cost and Utilization Project (HCUP), a partnership to inform decision making at all levels of government.[9] All inpatient discharges are collected and abstracted into a uniform format so that one massive database can be created for a participating state. Clinical and non-clinical information is collected from all patients regardless of insurance or lack thereof. It's a big undertaking with big gains to be had. We only used the 2007 SID of California for this chapter. Some of the more than 100 variables include:

- Patient demographics
- Patient location
- Principal and secondary diagnoses and procedures
- Admission and discharge dates and types
- Length of stay
- Days in intensive care or cardiac care
- Insurance and charges

The SID of California and Open Data

A data use agreement has to be signed in order to access the SID, and some amount of de-identification has already been performed on the data. Just the same, it might be useful to have a public version that could be used to train students, prepare research protocols, confirm published results, improve data quality, and who knows what else. For more precise analyses, the SID could be requested in more detail. The public version would be, well, public, so anyone could use the data as fast as they could download it. But as a public data release, the assumption of approximate complete knowledge would be appropriate to use.

We consider only a subset of the data available in the SID for California, shown in Table 4-1, to get an idea of how these assumptions work in practice. We're particularly interested in the level 2 quasi-identifiers—i.e., the longitudinal data—which in this case is the admission year, days since last service, and length of stay.

Table 4-1. Quasi-identifiers requested by researcher

Level	Field	Description
1	Gender	Patient's gender
1	BirthYear	Patient's year of birth
2	AdmissionYear	Year the patient was first admitted
2	DaysSinceLastService	Number of days since the patient's last medical service
2	LengthOfStay	Number of days the patient was in the hospital

Discharge abstracts are longitudinal, but most patients will only have one or two visits, which means only one or two rows of data per patient. Figure 4-4 captures this best, with a max number of visits of only 34. Of course, a patient that is very sick can have a very long length of stay, but this won't be captured in the number of visits. Rather, the information for the patient's stay will be in columns provided in the SID. In "Long Tails" on page 80 we'll see a very different form of longitudinal data, in which each medical claim is captured by a row (so that a long length of stay translates into many rows of data).

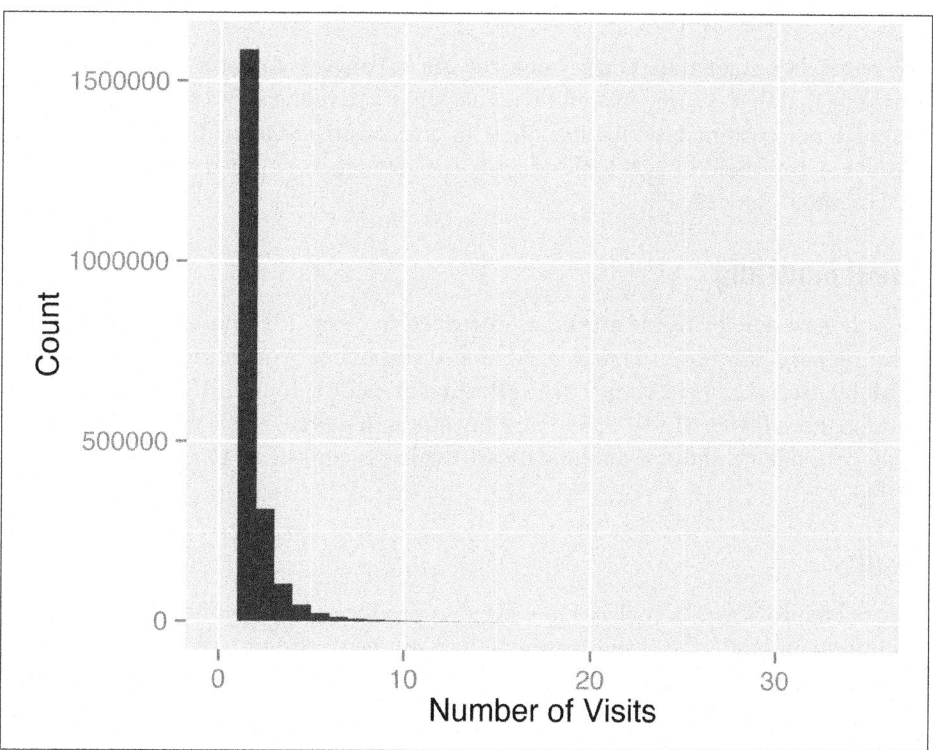

Figure 4-4. The short tail of discharge abstracts for the SID of California

The situation is similar to our example using BORN data (see "BORN Data Set" on page 52), except we're using longitudinal data here. We can't generalize the gender variable, but a generalization hierarchy was defined for each of the other variables, shown in Table 4-2. Notice that we're using top and bottom coding in our generalization hierarchy. A bottom code of 1910- for BirthYear means that any year strictly less than 1910 is grouped into "1910-." These top and bottom codes were necessary due to the distribution of data (it's never a good idea to blindly apply generalizations to data without first taking a look at it).

Table 4-2. Generalization hierarchy for the quasi-identifiers

Field	Generalization hierarchy
BirthYear	Bottom code 1910-: Year → 5-year interval → 10-year interval
AdmissionYear	Bottom code 2006-: 1-year interval → 2-year interval
DaysSinceLastService	Days up to six, week afterwards, top code 182+ → bottom code 7-, 28-day interval afterwards, top code 182+
LengthOfStay	Connected as to DaysSinceLastService

Risk Assessment

Any researcher, student, or comic book guy can have access to public data. So we have to assume that there's someone out there that will try to re-identify a record in the data. But we're not creating a public use file with any sensitive information, so let's set an overall risk threshold of 0.09 to de-identify the data set, as outlined in "Step 2: Setting the Threshold" on page 25.

Threat Modeling

We only have one plausible attack, as described in "Step 3: Examining Plausible Attacks" on page 26, and it requires us to look at the risk of re-identification in the data set all by itself (i.e., *Pr*(attempt) = 1, *Pr*(acquaintance) = 1, and *Pr*(breach) = 1). We therefore have *Pr*(re-id) ≤ 0.09, and nothing more. In this case we'll use maximum risk since we're talking about a public data set (which is equivalent to *k*-anonymity with $k = 11$).

Results

We used approximate complete knowledge to produce a de-identified data set with a minimized amount of cell suppression. Given our generalization hierarchy, the result was a data set with BirthYear bottom code 1910- with 5-year interval, AdmissionYear unchanged, DaysSinceLastService bottom code 7- with 28-day interval and top code 182+, and LengthOfStay the same as DaysSinceLastService because they were connected as QI to QI. Missingness and entropy are shown in Table 4-3 (these are the same measures we first saw in "Information Loss Metrics" on page 35). The results are a first step and can be improved on, as we'll see in subsequent chapters, but we somewhat expected this given how conservative the assumptions are (with an adversary that knows virtually everything about you… yikes).

Table 4-3. First attempt at de-identification

	Cell missingness	Record missingness	Entropy
Before	0.05%	3.14%	
After	15.3%	28.5%	44.7%

We also saw the binary/transactional approach in panel (d) of Figure 4-1, which isn't actually for longitudinal data but will produce a data set that is properly *k*-anonymized. As a baseline it will, admittedly, be excessive in its de-identification, but it's the only viable option for dealing with longitudinal health data under our current set of assumptions. Using approximate complete knowledge on the SID for California, the improvement in entropy was 71.3% compared to this baseline. So we're getting better, and we'll look at another adversary model that relaxes these assumptions even further when we get to Chapter 6.

Final Thoughts

Methods developed to de-identify cross-sectional data sets are not appropriate for use on longitudinal data sets. But longitudinal data sets are challenging to de-identify because there can be a lot of information in them. Assuming the adversary knows all will result in de-identified data sets that lose a tremendous amount of their utility. Reasonable assumptions about what an adversary can know need to be made. We've discussed some in this chapter, and we have more to come in subsequent chapters. Our purpose here was to get you started on the methods that are needed to deal with more complex data sets.

References

1. Schoenman J, Sutton J, Kintala S, Love D, Maw R: "The Value of Hospital Discharge Databases", Agency for Healthcare Research and Quality, 2005.

2. S. Hooley and l. Sweeney: "Survey of Publicly Available State Health Databases". Harvard University, 2013.

3. Robertson J.: "States' Hospital Data for Sale Puts Privacy in Jeopardy". Bloomberg News. June 5, 2013.

4. B. Malin, L. Sweeney, E. Newton, "Trail Re-identification: Learning Who You Are From Where You Have Been" (Pittsburgh, PA: Carnegie Mellon University, 2003).

5. B. Malin and L. Sweeney, "How (Not) to Protect Genomic Data Privacy in a Distributed Network: Using Trails Re-identification to Evaluate and Design Anonymity Protection Systems," *Journal of Biomedical Informatics* 37:3 (2004): 179–192.

6. Y. Xu, K. Wang, A. Fu, and P. Yu, "Anonymizing Transaction Databases for Publication," *IEEE Transactions on Knowledge Discovery and Data Mining* 23:(2008): 161–174.

7. G. Ghinita, Y. Tao, and P. Kalnis, "On the Anonymization of Sparse High-Dimensional Data," *Proceedings of the IEEE International Conference on Data Engineering* (ICDE, 2008).

8. C. Aggarwal, "On *k*-Anonymity and the Curse of Dimensionality," *Proceedings of the 31st International Conference on Very Large Data Bases* (VLDB Endowment, 2005).

9. Healthcare Cost and Utilization Project (HCUP) State Inpatient Databases (SID) (*http://1.usa.gov/sid-overview*)

CHAPTER 5

Dates, Long Tails, and Correlation: Insurance Claims Data

Insurance claims data represents a treasure trove of health information for all manner of analytics and research. In it you can find diagnostic and treatment information, details on providers used, and a great deal regarding finance and billing. The data is very precise, due to the need for precise accounting of medical charges and reimbursements, but it's primarily administrative data, which can pose all kinds of data cleaning and formatting problems. More importantly for our purposes, however, is that it can also present some unique challenges to de-identification that you wouldn't necessarily see in data collected primarily for research.

The Heritage Provider Network (HPN) presented us with a unique challenge: to de-identify a large claims data set, with up to three-year longitudinal patient profiles, for an essentially public data release. This work motivated a lot of the methods we present here. The methods are useful whenever you deal with longitudinal data, but especially when there are a large number of observations per patient.

The Heritage Health Prize

The Heritage Provider Network is a provider of health care services in California. They initiated the Heritage Health Prize (HHP) competition to develop a predictive algorithm that can "identify patients who will be admitted to a hospital within the next year using historical claims data."[1] The data provided to competitors consisted of up to three years' worth of data for some 113,000 patients, comprising a total 2,668,990 claims. The competition ran from 2011-04 to 2013-04, with a potential reward of $3,000,000 for the best algorithm. We'll use data from the HHP, before de-identification and subsampling, to describe the methods presented in this chapter.

Date Generalization

Insurance claims will undoubtedly have dates: the date of service, when drugs were dispensed, or when specimens were collected. Knowing a sequence of dates gives an adversary a way to re-identify individuals. For example, if a relative or neighbor knows that you had surgery on Tuesday, a claim for anesthesia on Tuesday would definitely be consistent with your surgery. Multiple surgery-related charges on Tuesday would further strengthen the evidence that this was your health record.

This might seem like a stretch—obviously a lot of people would have had surgery that day—but it's an important piece of information that has to be included in the risk assessment. The more quasi-identifiers you have in a data set, the more unique patients become. And keep in mind that a pseudonym is used to link patient information across claims in a de-identified data set, so these sequences of dates are not lost.

It's also reasonable to assume that acquaintances, at the very least, will know the precise (or general) date for health care services. The example of a neighbor is a good one, but so is a co-worker or a friend. And people talk, so word gets around, especially if the treatment is for something serious (like the treatment for a major illness, or a major surgery). It's even worse for famous people, as the information will be spread by the media and stored in print and online.

Randomizing Dates Independently of One Another

A simple way to de-identify date information is to add noise to each date (essentially shifting each date independently of one another). If the noise added is from a Gaussian or Laplace distribution, it leaves open opportunities for attacking the data using modeling techniques that can average out the noise. It's therefore better to generate the noise from a uniform distribution. We could, for example, randomly shift each date by up to 15 days in either direction (earlier or later).

Consider a situation where a patient named Bob has a unique pattern of dates that results in a high risk of re-identification. Maybe Bob was seeking care during a prolonged length of time, making him stand out. Randomizing dates independently of one another, adding or subtracting up to 15 days as in Table 5-1, makes the dates of his claims fall into the same range of uncertainty as those of every other patient in the data.

Table 5-1. Date sequence for Bob's medical claims, randomized by +/– 15 days

Original sequence	Randomized
2001/04/08	2001/04/23
2002/05/07	2002/05/18
2002/08/12	2002/08/06
2003/07/27	2003/07/29
2003/08/11	2003/07/28

Adding noise to dates could, however, distort the order of claims by date, as was the case for the last two dates in Table 5-1. We could end up with a claim for post-op recovery charges being dated before the surgery itself, which wouldn't make much sense (or might make you think the health care provider is doing some seriously funky stuff). Another example would be admission and discharge dates. Randomizing these dates independently of one another could result in a patient discharge before admission—although that may sound like good medicine, it doesn't make much sense!

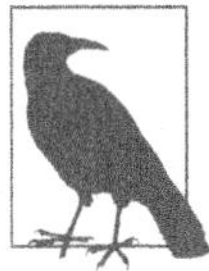

Generally speaking, de-identification should produce data that still makes sense, or analysts won't trust it. Of course, they'll probably be used to seeing "bad data," with all sorts of formatting and data problems, but de-identification shouldn't make this worse. Cleaning data is not the purview of de-identification, but maintaining its integrity should be.

What maintaining the integrity of a data set really means depends on the type of analysis that's needed. In some cases the exact order of events won't matter, just the general trend —maybe monthly, or seasonal, or even yearly for summary statistics and frequency plots. If a health care facility wants to run some statistics on admissions for the past year, randomizing dates to within a month won't matter, even if some discharges come before admissions.

Shifting the Sequence, Ignoring the Intervals

Another approach that might seem to make sense—in order to preserve the order of claims by date—is to shift the whole sequence of dates for a patient so that the order of claims is preserved. In Table 5-2 all dates for Bob's health care claims have been shifted by –15 days. We still used a random number between –15 and 15, from a uniform distribution, but this time the same value was applied to all dates in order to preserve their order.

Table 5-2. Date sequence for Bob's medical claims, shifted

Original sequence	Shifted sequence
2001/04/08	2001/03/24
2002/05/07	2002/04/22
2002/08/12	2002/07/28
2003/07/27	2003/07/12
2003/08/11	2003/07/27

The problem with this approach is that the intervals between dates are preserved exactly. So even if you don't recognize the dates, you could look at the intervals and determine when they match Bob's health claims. If the dates can be known, so can the intervals between them (an easy and direct inference). The sequence of intervals may even be easier to recognize than the dates for treatments that have a known pattern, like dialysis treatments or chemotherapy. We didn't have to worry about this when we randomized dates because when the end points are unknown, so are the intervals between them.

What if there are unusually large intervals between claims? In Table 5-2, the interval between Bob's first two claims is maintained at 394 days. This could stand out among other records in the data set. Bob could be the only 55-year-old male with an interval of more than 365 days in the database. Of course, we have to treat dates as longitudinal, so the intervals would be considered using a longitudinal risk assessment. But the point is that the intervals themselves pose a re-identification risk, and must therefore be managed somehow. So shifting a sequence of dates is not an approach we recommend.

Generalizing Intervals to Maintain Order

A better approach that can be used to protect claims while maintaining their order by date is to generalize the intervals between them. To provide a data set with dates, instead of intervals, we can use the first (randomized) date in the claim sequence as an anchor and add a random value from the generalized intervals to all subsequent claims.

Let's go through this process step by step, again using Bob's sequence of dates. In Table 5-3 we converted the original sequence to intervals between claims, with the first date kept as the anchor.

Table 5-3. Date sequence for Bob's medical claims converted to intervals

Original sequence	Converted sequence
2001/04/08	2001/04/08
2002/05/07	394 days
2002/08/12	97 days
2003/07/27	349 days
2003/08/11	15 days

Next we generalized the converted sequence. Following our previous examples, we generalized the first date, our anchor, to month, as shown in Table 5-4. But many analysts don't want to deal with generalized dates, so we then randomized the intervals, as we did for dates (i.e., selecting an integer at random from the generalized interval). Since the anchor is generalized to month, all subsequent dates will also be randomized to within a month. But we needed to do something with the intervals, or else we'd have the same problems as before. So, we generalized them to within a week.

Table 5-4. Date sequence for Bob's medical claims as de-identified intervals

Converted sequence	Generalized sequence	Randomized
2001/04/08	2001/04	2001/04/23
394 days	[393-399]	398 days
97 days	[92-98]	96 days
349 days	[344-350]	345 days
15 days	[15-21]	20 days

Finally, we converted the intervals back to dates by adding each randomized interval to the previous date, with the generalized anchor date providing the starting point, as shown in Table 5-5. Because we added the intervals between dates to the previous dates in the sequence, we guaranteed that the order of claims was maintained, as well as the approximate distances between them in time.

Table 5-5. Date sequence for Bob's medical claims de-identified

Original sequence	Intermediate step	De-identified sequence
2001/04/08	2001/04/23	2001/04/23
2002/05/07	2001/04/23 + 398 days	2002/05/26
2002/08/12	2002/05/26 + 96 days	2002/08/30
2003/07/27	2002/08/30 + 345 days	2003/08/10
2003/08/11	2003/08/10 + 20 days	2003/08/30

If admission and discharge dates were included in the claims data, they would be included as quasi-identifiers for each visit. We could calculate length of stay and time since last service, then apply the same approach just shown to de-identify these values.

Rather than generalizing all the date intervals to the same level (global recoding), as we've described, we could instead generalize intervals specifically based on need for each record (local recoding). For example, for patients in large equivalence classes with much lower risk of re-identification, perhaps the date intervals could be five days long instead of the seven days we used. Normally when generalizing information this is bad, because you end up with inconsistent formats between records (e.g., one record with interval "[1-5]," and another with "[1-7]"). But in this case we're only using the generalization to determine the interval from which we'll draw a random number, so in the end the dates have the same format (day, month, year). The point would be to decrease information loss, at the expense of some computational overhead.

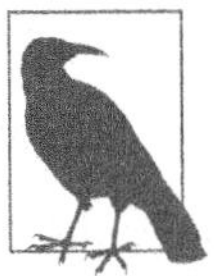

The generalization for the anchor date and intervals should be given to data analysts. They may need this information to choose models and interpret results. As a simple example, if the date were generalized to weeks, the analysts would know that their results would be accurate to within a week at best. If some form of local recoding were used to de-identify the data set, then they would need to know the equivalent generalization under global recoding (or the max generalization used under local recoding, which would be the same).

Dates and Intervals and Back Again

We don't want to lose sight of the fact that the intervals between dates were derived from, well, dates. If we drop the anchor, or reorder the intervals before generalizing, then we've lost the original dates. That would be bad for de-identification, because dates of service are quasi-identifiers, plain and simple. We need this information to do a proper risk assessment. Not only that, but there's information contained in the pattern of dates you don't want to lose. The sequence of intervals (4 months, 3 months, 2 months, 1 month) might represent a patient that's getting worse, whereas the sequence of intervals (1 month, 2 months, 3 months, 4 months) might represent a patient that's getting better. The point here is that the anchor date and the order of the intervals need to be preserved during the risk assessment, and during de-identification.

When we sample random interval values from generalized intervals, note that we aren't using the original dates (or intervals) any longer. You have two dates in the same generalized interval? Then sample two random values in the generalized interval! It doesn't matter what values are returned (if they're ordered or unordered), because they're added sequentially so that the order of events is preserved. This is very different from the scenario in which we randomized the original dates by +/–15 days.

Now you might worry that generalizing intervals (e.g., going from days to seven-day intervals), then adding it all up at the end to produce a new sequence of dates, might skew the sequence to be much longer than the original. But because we're drawing the sample from a uniform distribution, we expect the mean to be the center of the interval's range. It's reasonable to assume that the dates are randomly distributed among the intervals—i.e., they're drawn from a statistical distribution. Therefore, when we add up the randomized intervals, the last interval of the sequence is expected to be within the final generalized interval for the patient.

Now, if there's bias in the dates (e.g., they're always at the start of the month), it's possible that when the dates are added up the final dates will get pushed outside this range. For example, generalizing to seven-day intervals, on average we expect that the sequence (1, 8, 15) would be randomized to (4, 11, 19). The original intervals sum up to 24 days whereas the randomized intervals sum up to 34 days, which means the final date would be off by 10 days. No big deal if your anchor date was generalized to month, but do that for 20 visits and the bias grows significantly.

This raises another important point—what about consecutive days in hospital? Intervals of one day, because of an overnight stay, can't be changed to intervals greater than one day. Not only would this greatly bias the final date if the patient has had many days in hospital, but it breaks the cardinal rule of not producing data that doesn't make sense! Thus, we would keep consecutive visits together, and randomize the intervals between visits starting from two days and onwards.

A Different Anchor

When we have records for infants or children in a data set, date generalization can produce dates of service that are before the date of birth. Say an infant is born on 2012/01/15, and generalized to within a year of that date in the process of de-identification. Maybe the new anonymized date of birth is now 2012/07/23. Now say the infant's first date of service in the data set is 2012/01/18. If the anchor date were generalized to month, the first date of service would end up being before the date of birth. This would of course be very confusing to anyone analyzing the data.

What we need to do, then, is use the date of birth as the anchor and compute the first interval from the date of birth rather than from the first date of service for the patient. That way the order is preserved with respect to the date of birth.

A similar situation arises with the date of death. We don't want to have a date of service that occurs after the date of death. Where there's a date of death, we would therefore add that at the end of the sequence so that it's calculated based on the interval from the last date of service. This way we can ensure order consistency for start and end of life anchors.

Other Quasi-Identifiers

Let's not forget that there are other quasi-identifiers to deal with. We mentioned this at the outset, but it bears repeating. Randomizing dates or intervals between dates won't hide the exact diseases or surgeries reported. Say Bob is the only person in the data set that has had appendicitis in the first half of 2001. Shifting dates by a month or two won't change this. So we need to include dates as part of the risk assessment, even though we've simplified our discussion by ignoring other quasi-identifiers.

As with any quasi-identifier, the generalization of dates needs to be done in the context of other quasi-identifiers, and with a well-defined generalization hierarchy (e.g., days, weeks, months). But dates are longitudinal, and managing the risk from the sequence, or even the set, of dates for a patient can be challenging. If we increase the level of generalization we may seriously deteriorate the quality of the data. Although we did point out that it depends on what analyses will be done with the data, at some point the level of generalization will cross the border into Crazy Town. It's the trade-off between re-identification risk and data quality.

Consider a situation where Bob has a unique pattern of dates that results in a high risk of re-identification. During the period when Bob was seeking care, no one else in his age group and ZIP code was also seeking care. Sure, there were people going to see their health care providers now and again, but Bob had persistent problems requiring medical treatment. This makes him stand out, because dates are longitudinal quasi-identifiers. The only way to reduce the risk of re-identification for Bob would be to increase the level of generalization of the quasi-identifiers in the data set, or suppress dates.

Another point worth considering is that some of these other quasi-identifiers may be used to infer dates. What if a certain procedure was only introduced at a certain point in time, maybe on 2010-04-01? An adversary with the right smarts might see this procedure appear in Bob's records on 2010-01-01 and know they can subtract three months from all the dates! This sort of attack might work if all the dates were moved by the same amount, but it's less likely to succeed when the intervals between events have been modified. It does, however, call into question the effectiveness of major changes (say of mulitple months) to the overall sequence. Perhaps unlikely, but worth keeping in mind.

Connected Dates

The concept of connected fields is also important when we deal with dates. Sometimes we see dates in a claim that are so highly correlated that we need to treat them as connected variables. For example, there may be a date of service and a log date that indicates when the information was entered into the electronic medical record. The log date will almost always be on the same day as the day of service.

We can't ignore such connections because it's easy to infer the correct date of service from the log date. So it's necessary to shift the log date by the same amount as the date of service. This ensures data consistency and eliminates the possibility of an inappropriate inference.

Another example, to drive the point home, is the start date of a treatment plan, and the dates the treatments are administered. These would be two connected quasi-identifiers. And how about a log date of when information was entered into the system, and a log date of any modifications to the record? These would be two connected dates, but not quasi-identifiers. However, they would need to be connected to the quasi-identifier dates just described! Yikes, this is getting complicated—but it's the reality of working with health data, which can be as complicated as you can imagine.

Long Tails

Now let's move on to a property of claims data that can pose a unique challenge to the de-identification of a data set. We know that claims data is longitudinal, but most patients will only have a handful of health care visits. Those that have severe or chronic conditions will undoubtedly have more than a handful of claims, because they'll have more visits, interventions, or treatments. But then there will be some that have even *more* claims, because they are extreme cases.

It's important to understand that every procedure and drug, even medical supplies and transportation, has an associated charge. Insurance data tracks mundane things like giving the patient an aspirin, or anesthesia, or an ambulance ride. During a single visit, there may be tens of charges, and each will be captured in a row of data.

The result of this wide range of patients, and their resulting claims, is well demonstrated in Figure 5-1. This is the long tail of claims data, driven by the very sick. All together, there were 5,426,238 claims in this data set, for 145,650 patients. The vast majority of patients had less than 10 claims—but some had more than 1,300 claims.

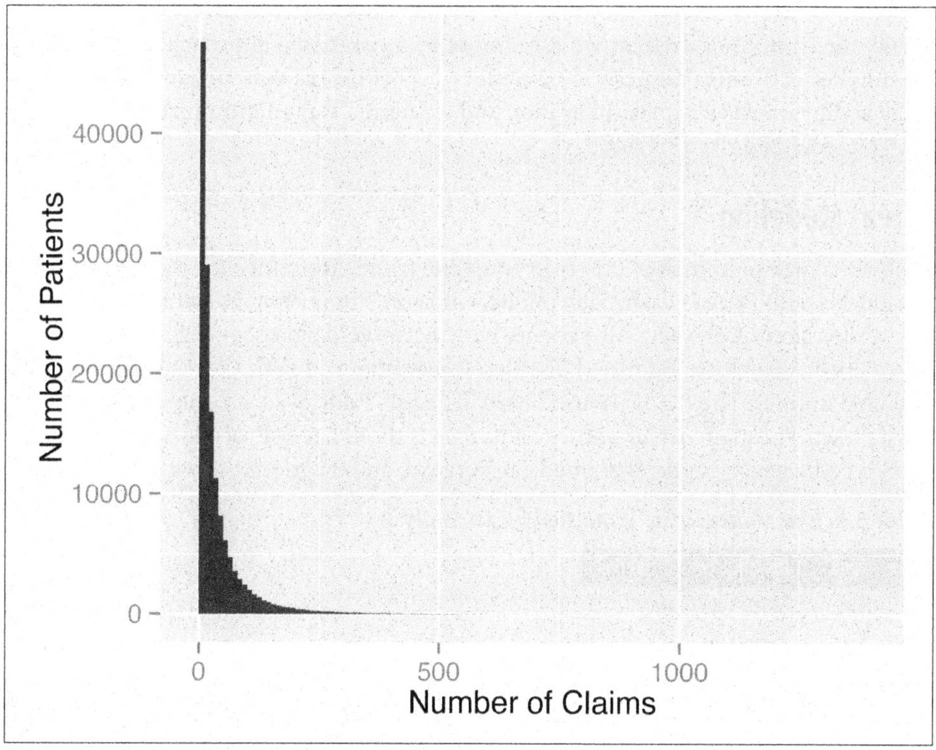

Figure 5-1. The long tail of claims data for HPN

The Risk from Long Tails

An adversary might know the number of claims that a patient has had, or at least the range. It's the patients in the long tail of the distribution who are most at risk. All an adversary needs to know is that they have some lower bound in the number of claims —if that lower bound is high enough, the number of patients in that category will be quite low. Say an adversary knows someone has been through a lot of procedures during multiple hospital stays, or one very long hospital visit. The adversary doesn't need to know the exact number of procedures, but may be able to accurately guess it was over 1,000. Combining that information with basic demographics results in only a handful of patients per equivalence class.

To protect against such attacks, we could cut the tail of that distribution at, say, the 95th or 99th percentile. At the 95th percentile, patients with more than 139 claims would have claims truncated (those above 139), resulting in the removal of 11% of claims; at the 99th percentile, patients with more than 266 claims would have claims truncated (those above 266), resulting in the removal of 2.8% of claims. That's a lot of claims to remove from the data set for an ad hoc method that hasn't factored risk into the approach.

Ideally the truncation method we use should be a risk-based approach and minimize the number of claims that need to be removed. That means that the number of claims needs to be treated as a quasi-identifier, and we need a way to minimize truncation to meet a predefined risk threshold.

Threat Modeling

We'll use a maximum risk of 0.1 to demonstrate truncation, since the data set from the Heritage Health Prize is essentially public, with some important constraints, and a low risk of invasion of privacy. All patients with sensitive diagnoses—e.g., mental health disorders or sexually transmitted diseases—were removed with exact definitions documented online.[2] The fields we used here, listed in Table 5-6, are only a subset of the full data set. The main driver of the claims data is the Current Procedural Terminology (CPT)[3] code, which captures all medical, surgical, and diagnostic services.[4]

Table 5-6. Quasi-identifiers requested by an analyst

Level	Field	Description
1	Age	Patient's age in years
1	Sex	Patient's sex
2	CPTCode	CPT code for the claim
2	Date	Date of service for the claim

Number of Claims to Truncate

An adversary is very unlikely to know the exact number of claims that a patient has in a data set. For the HHP data set we assumed that an adversary would know the number of claims to within a range of 5. So, if a patient had exactly 14 claims, the adversary would only know that it was somewhere in the range of 11 to 15, but not that it was exactly 14.

This assumption is quite conservative—in practice we could use a range of 10 claims. We could also add a cutoff at 500 claims, so that the adversary would just know that the patient had more than 500 claims, but not the exact number. For a public data release we might prefer to be conservative, so we'll carry on with the assumption of accuracy to within five claims.

We divide the number of claims into a series of bins. Each bin is a discrete interval of the number of claims a patient can have, with a range of five claims each. We sort these in increasing order and count the number of patients in each bin. The result is a frequency table, shown in Table 5-7. This is just an example based on a subset of the HPN data—the original HPN data is simply too large for demonstration purposes.

Table 5-7. Frequency table for the number of claims

Number of claims	Number of patients
[1-5]	100
[6-10]	50
[11-15]	40
[16-20]	30
[21-25]	7
[26-30]	4
[31-35]	11

With a maximum risk threshold of 0.1, we don't want the number of patients in a bin (determined by the number of claims) to be less than 10. In other words, we're treating the number of claims as a quasi-identifier, and we've generalized the number of claims so that they're only considered within a range of five claims.

The truncation algorithm works backward, from the last bin, with the highest number of claims ([31-35]), to the first bin, with the lowest number of claims ([1-5]). We look at the number of patients in a bin, and if it doesn't meet our risk threshold, we move those patients up to the next bin by removing some of their claims. Let's walk through an example.

There are 11 patients with [31-35] claims. This number is larger than the minimum bin size for a maximum risk threshold of 0.1, so we leave it as is. Next, there are four patients with [26-30] claims. Here we have a problem, so we "move" these patients to the next bin upwards, the [21-25] bin. We do this by removing claims for these four patients so that they have between 21 and 25 claims. The exact number of claims they'll end up with will be randomly chosen from the range [21-25].

By doing this, we've added four new patients to the [21-25] bin. After that movement, there are now 11 patients in the [21-25] bin, which makes it large enough for the 0.1 threshold. The remaining bins are also large enough, so we're done truncating claims.

This binning approach allowed us to minimize the amount of truncation to only 0.06% of claims in the HHP data set. Contrast that with the 11% and 2.6% of claims that were truncated using 95th and 99th percentiles, respectively. Not to mention that we hadn't treated the number of claims as a quasi-identifier in the percentile method!

Which Claims to Truncate

So how do we decide which claims to truncate? To reduce the risk of re-identification, we want to remove claims with the rarest values on the quasi-identifiers. For the HHP data set, the level 2 quasi-identifiers we're concerned with are the date and CPT code. If a person has a claim with a rare procedure, that claim is a good candidate for truncation because the rare procedure makes that claim, and therefore that person, stand out.

The number of people with a particular quasi-identifier value is called its *support*. The lower the support, the more that quasi-identifier value stands out, and the higher the risk of re-identification is for the people with that value. We could sort claims by their support for CPT codes, for example, and truncate those with the lowest support to reach our desired level of truncation.

A rare CPT code could, however, be coupled with a very common disease. That creates a conflict, because now we have to decide whether a claim is a good candidate for truncation or not. One way to resolve this conflict is to consider the variability in the support for the set of quasi-identifiers in a particular claim. If a claim has a low mean support but some quasi-identifiers with relatively high support, the claim has *high variability*. But if a claim has a low mean support and all its quasi-identifiers have relatively low support, the claim has *low variability*. Obviously, the low-variability claims should be truncated before the high-variability ones.

To capture these factors, we define a score based on the mean support, adjusted by the variability in support. The point of the score is to capture events that are the most rare among the claims, and therefore single out the best candidates for truncation. The basic calculation is pretty straightforward: first we compute the support for each quasi-identifier in a claim, and then we compute the mean (μ) and standard deviation (σ) of the support values. From this we derive an equation that linearizes this relationship, from a mean support of 1 to the max support. Two examples are shown in Figure 5-2: low variability and high variability. Next, we order claims by score and truncate those with the lowest scores first.

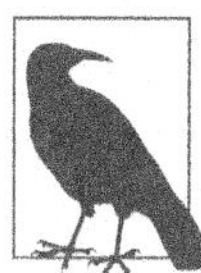

Because it's a bit messy, we've included the equation we use in Figure 5-2. Although this isn't a book of equations, we felt that this time it was warranted. Please forgive us.

In order to get a score that ranges from 0 to 1 for all events, we need to scale our linear equation with the max standard deviation (σ_{max}) and max support (sup_{max}). The max support could be the max number of patients in the data set (a quick and dirty solution), or the max support across all quasi-identifiers for all of a patient's claims.

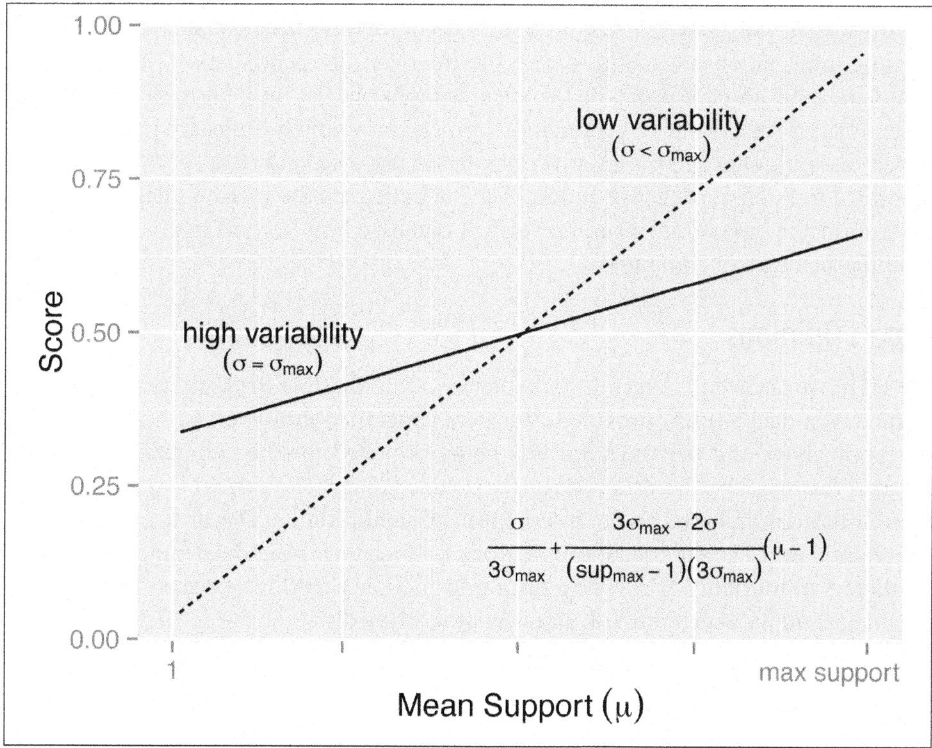

Figure 5-2. Balancing support with variability to find claims to truncate

With this scheme we can minimize the amount of truncation, and truncate only the claims that are most identifying. In practice, truncation is effective for claims data or other transactional data where the number of claims or transactions per patient is large. A plot of the number of claims or transactions in a data set that shows a long tail is a clear indication that truncation would be appropriate.

Correlation of Related Items

One major issue to consider when de-identifying detailed medical information is the correlation among variables. De-identifying a data set may not be effective if other quasi-identifiers can be inferred from the data. For example, let's say that we're disclosing only basic demographics and prescription drug information. There's no diagnosis information in the data set at all. Without the diagnosis information, we may believe that the risk of re-identification is very small. But can an adversary use the demographics and drug information to predict the missing diagnosis information? If that's the case, the predicted diagnosis information could potentially increase the re-identification risk significantly.

Unfortunately, the answer turns out to be a qualified yes—an adversary could predict missing information and compromise the intended de-identification. An adversary could ask a health care professional, such as a pharmacist, to determine the missing diagnosis information. It's a pharmacist's job to know which drugs are prescribed for which diseases, after all. Or an adversary could use a second data set that is not de-identified to build a predictive model that can anticipate the missing diagnosis information. In the case of an insurance claims database, this second data set could, for example, belong to a competitor.

Expert Opinions

For HHP, we needed to determine whether or not to disclose drug information on top of the claim data already provided. We were concerned, however, with inferences of diagnosis above and beyond what was being provided for the competition data set. Because this was a public data release, the detailed diagnosis codes (of which there are literally thousands, based on the International Classification of Diseases, or ICD[5]) were generalized into 45 primary condition groups, which have been determined to be good predictors of mortality.[6] Providing drug information would have risked breaking the generalization on which our risk assessment was based!

To illustrate this, we conducted a simple experiment with 31 Ontario pharmacists. Pharmacists are trained to determine drugs for specific diagnoses and, to a certain extent, the reverse as well. So they're in a good position to provide extra information about, or predict, diagnoses from drug profiles. We gave each pharmacist longitudinal data on 20 patients, with their basic demographics and generic drugs that they took. They were asked to predict each patient's primary condition group, ICD chapter, and three-digit ICD code (i.e., increasing the level of detail at each step). Their success rates are shown in Table 5-8.

Table 5-8. Accuracy of pharmacists in predicting diseases from drugs

	Primary condition	ICD chapter	Three-digit ICD
Accuracy	0.622	0.381	0.323

The pharmacists did a decent job at predicting the primary condition, but less so when they had to predict the ICD chapter and three-digit ICD-9 code. However, if the intention was not to provide any kind of diagnosis information, their ability to predict the primary condition could still increase the re-identification risk of the patients above the assumed levels, and above the threshold used. Of course, you don't have to go to this extent and conduct your own experiments when de-identifying data sets. But you should ask experts their opinions about what information can be inferred from the data you intend to release.

Predictive Models

Another approach we've used is to build predictive models to test what information can be reasonably inferred from a de-identified data set. This can identify sources of risk, but only if you believe an adversary can have access to a data set similar to yours, prior to de-identification.

For HHP, we used machine learning models to predict detailed diagnoses (based on ICD codes) using the other information in the claims data set, including the primary condition groups. We divided the HPN data set into 40 different subsets, each representing a primary condition group. In total, we used 1,458,420 claims, with an average of 36,450 claims per subset. They had attributes that described a patient's personal profile, including hospitalization, laboratory tests, and prescribed drug codes, which were used to predict the ICD-9 code of the patient.

For each subset we computed the proportion (percentage) of claims that were correctly classified into the three-digit ICD-9 code by the machine learning algorithm. For comparison purposes, we used as the baseline the assignment of the most frequent diagnosis code. That way we could evaluate how much better the machine learning model was compared to a simple guess based on a majority rule. The results are shown in Table 5-9. For a simple machine learning algorithm, the Naive Bayes classifier, predictions were better than the baseline for 32 of the 40 primary condition groups.

Table 5-9. Accuracy of machine learning models in predicting diseases from HHP data

Accuracy	Three-digit ICD	Five-digit ICD
Baseline	0.428	0.273
Machine learning	0.654	0.506

Implications for De-Identifying Data Sets

The results of these analyses, both the expert predictions and the learning models, had an impact on the level of detail of the drug data that was disclosed as part of HHP. Since many organizations get patient claims data, it seemed plausible that an adversary could seek the help of an expert or build an accurate model to predict more detailed diagnosis information than was included in the competition data set.

The bottom line is that you must be careful of correlated information in medical data. There are plausible inference channels from one part of the data to another. This means that if you generalize or suppress one part of the record, you need to verify that other information in the record cannot be used to impute or provide details that undo the de-identification. You can do this by running modeling experiments similar to the ones described here.

Final Thoughts

There's a lot of information in claims data, and a lot that needs to be done for de-identification. The data will contain dates, and those dates will be longitudinal. Analysts usually want to work with the day, month, and year of real dates. Generalizing dates and providing a random date from the generalization works, but may mix up the order of claims. Converting to intervals between dates, while maintaining an anchor and their order, provides a simple yet effective way to de-identify dates while preserving the order of events.

A bigger challenge with claims data is the enormous number of claims some patients may have—our so-called "long tail." Treating the number of claims as a quasi-identifier, with a predefined level of precision, allows you to incorporate this risk into the de-identification process. Truncating claims allows you to manage this risk, and our support-based approach allows the number of truncated claims to be minimized so as little information is lost as possible.

Probably the biggest unknown, however, is the risk from correlation. For this we need to talk to medical experts to determine what can be learned from the data we want to disclose. We simply can't assume that withholding data elements will prevent their disclosure. If drugs are going to be included in a released data set, you might want to include diseases in the risk assessment. And if you're going to provide detailed information for some data elements, think hard about whether or not it can be used to infer beyond the generalizations provided elsewhere. If you can, build your own predictive models to test your assumptions!

References

1. Heritage Provider Network Health Prize (*http://www.heritagehealthprize.com*)

2. K. El Emam, L. Arbuckle, G. Koru, B. Eze, L. Gaudette, E. Neri, S. Rose, J. Howard, and J. Gluck, "De-identification Methods for Open Health Data: The Case of the Heritage Health Prize Claims Dataset," *Journal of Medical Internet Research* 14:1 (2012): e33.

3. CPT is a registered trademark of the American Medical Association.

4. American Medical Association, *CPT 2006 Professional Edition (CPT/Current Procedural Terminology (Professional Edition))*. (Chicago, IL: AMA Press, 2005).

5. World Health Organization/Centers for Disease Control and Prevention. *International Classification of Diseases, Ninth Revision, Clinical Modification (ICD-9-CM)* (*http://1.usa.gov/icd9-mod*).

6. G.J. Escobar, J.D. Greene, P. Scheirer, M.N. Gardner, D. Draper, and P. Kipnis, "Risk-Adjusting Hospital Inpatient Mortality Using Automated Inpatient, Outpatient, and Laboratory Databases, *Medical Care* 46:3 (2008): 232–39.

CHAPTER 6
Longitudinal Events Data: A Disaster Registry

Complex health data sets contain information about patients over periods of time. A person's medical history can be taken as a series of events: when they were first diagnosed with a disease, when they received treatment, when they were admitted to an emergency department. Our case study for this chapter is the World Trade Center (WTC) disaster registry. The collapse of the Twin Towers at the World Trade Center is one of those unforgettable disasters that has deeply affected many people, both locally and abroad. The Clinical Center of Excellence at Mount Sinai has been following WTC workers and volunteers for years in an effort to provide them with the best treatment for the physical and mental health conditions related to their WTC service.[1] As the saying goes, you can't manage what you don't measure.

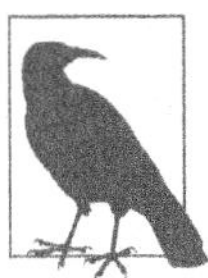

We'll be using the term "events" to refer to a patient's medical information in this discussion because of the structure of the WTC data. But the methods we explore here apply equally well to other data sets, such as discharge data or claims data. When we get to the methods themselves, we'll point out how they apply to these other scenarios, if the differences need to be highlighted.

In looking at this longitudinal disaster registry, we need to revisit the assumptions we make about what an adversary can know to re-identify patients in a data set. We started with an adversary that knows all, then relaxed some of our assumptions in Chapter 4 (an adversary can't know everything, or we might as well pack it in). What we need is a way to measure average risk when the adversary doesn't know all. What we need is the concept of *adversary power*.

Adversary Power

A patient can have multiple events related to a medical case, such as the multiple procedures the patient has undergone or diseases he has been diagnosed with. But it would be overly paranoid to assume that an adversary knows all of these things. The adversary may know that someone fainted and was admitted on a certain day, but know neither the diagnosis codes for everything the doctors wrote down about the patient, nor all the procedures performed.

So it's reasonable to assume that an adversary will have information on only a subset of these events. The amount of information the adversary has is known as the *power* of the adversary, and we use this idea to estimate the risk of re-identification. We don't know what type of adversary we might be dealing with, so we have to assume all of the plausible attacks described in "Measuring Risk Under Plausible Attacks" on page 29 (except for the public data release, which would require using maximum risk).

The power of the adversary reflects the number of events about which the adversary has some background information. It applies only to the longitudinal events (level 2) and not to the basic information about patients, like their demographics (level 1). This basic level 1 information about patients is assumed to be known, the same as it would be if we were working with a cross-sectional data set on its own (like we did in Chapter 3).

Now, if there's only one quasi-identifier in the level 2 events, the adversary power is the number of values that the adversary is assumed to know in that quasi-identifier. For example, if the quasi-identifier is the diagnosis code, the power is the number of diagnosis codes that the adversary knows.

A power of p therefore translates into p quasi-identifier values that can be used for re-identifying patients. If there's more than one quasi-identifier, the adversary power is the number of values that the adversary is assumed to know in *each* quasi-identifier. A power of p this time translates into p quasi-identifier values times the number of quasi-identifiers. So two quasi-identifiers means $2 \times p$ pieces of information that can be used by the adversary for re-identifying a patient.

So, if the date of diagnosis is one quasi-identifier and the diagnosis itself is another, the adversary would know the dates for p events and the diagnoses for another p events. The events might overlap, or they might not—it depends on how we decide to sample for adversary power (which we'll get to in "A Sample of Power" on page 94). But all in all, the adversary has $2 \times p$ pieces of background information for a patient.

Keeping Power in Check

Previous efforts that considered adversary power always assumed that the power was fixed for all patients.[2] But intuitively, it makes sense that the adversary would have different amounts of background knowledge for different patients. Everything else being equal, it's easier to have background information about a patient with a large number of events than about a patient with few events. Therefore, we expect power to increase with the number of events that a patient has undergone.

Also, it's likely that certain pieces of background information are more easily knowable than others by an adversary, making it necessary to treat the quasi-identifiers separately when it comes to computing adversary power. For example, it would be easier to know diagnosis values for patients with chronic conditions whose diagnoses keep repeating across visits than to know diagnosis values for patients who have a variety of different ailments.

Further, if the adversary knows the information in one visit, they can more easily predict the information in other visits, increasing the amount of background knowledge available for an attack. So, the diversity of values on a quasi-identifier across a patient's visits becomes an important consideration. And we therefore expect the power of an adversary to decrease with the diversity of values on the quasi-identifiers.

To capture these differences, we break patients into four groups, shown in Table 6-1. For patients with few medical events and high variability between those events, little background information will be available to an adversary, who consequently will have a lower level of adversary power. For patients with many medical events and low variability between those events, more background information will be available to an adversary, giving him a higher level of adversary power. The other combinations fall in between.

Table 6-1. I've got the power, oh Snap! Of course, the power values are just to illustrate relative size—this changes based on max power.

	Low variability	High variability
Few events	$p = 5$	$p = 3$
Many events	$p = 7$	$p = 5$

Power in Practice

We let p_{max} be the maximum power assumed of an adversary, n be the number of events for the patient, and v be the variability of the quasi-identifier for the patient. Then, for each patient, we calculate the adversary power for each quasi-identifier:

Adversary power for quasi-identifier (applied to a single patient)

$$p = \lceil 1 + (p_{max} - 1) \times (n / v) / \max_{patients}(n / v) \rceil$$

The max function is over all patients, because we want to scale adversary power based on the highest ratio of n over v. The variability v ranges from 0 for no variability (i.e., the quasi-identifier never changes value) to 1 for maximum variability (i.e., the quasi-identifier is always changing), and is a probability derived from the Simpson index.[3]

Just to explain the equation and the logic behind it a bit more, we start with a value of 1 in computing adversary power because we have to start somewhere. We don't want to assume that the adversary knows absolutely nothing about a patient! The rest of the equation involves scaling the range of power values, so that the adversary power goes from 1 to a max that we define, our so-called p_{max} (whereas everything else in the equation is determined from the data). We also round up (e.g., 1.1 becomes 2) so that we assume the adversary has more power rather than less.

Which brings us to an important question: what is the maximum possible power? For longitudinal data sets with multiple quasi-identifiers, we typically use a max power of 5 per quasi-identifier.[4] It's not uncommon for us to have anywhere between 5 and 10 quasi-identifiers to work with, which means a maximum power of anywhere from $5 \times 5 = 25$ to $5 \times 10 = 50$ pieces of background information about a single patient.

Oh great lobster in the sky, 50 pieces of background info about a single patient? That's a lot of medical information to know about someone! To think that this is less than knowing all of a patient's medical history really puts things into perspective—there can be a lot of information in longitudinal health data. That's why we're trying to scale back our assumptions to a more reasonable level of what an adversary could know.

A Sample of Power

We sample patients' quasi-identifier values so that we can use their background information to simulate an attack on the data. Typically we randomly sample from 1,000 to 5,000 patients in a data set, collect our sample of their background information, then see how many patients we can match to in the full data set. The proportion of unique matches out of our sample of patients is a form of average risk. We consider three ways to sample a patient's background information, and each has its pros and cons:

Random sample per quasi-identifier

This is a no-brainer. Random sampling is always the first approach when sampling. The problem with it in this case is that health data is always strongly correlated across records. A record can have multiple fields related to an event, and a patient can have many records in a longitudinal data set. If we have diseases in one column and procedures in another, a random sample of one may in fact imply the other. But since they are sampled independently of one another, we end up with twice the amount of information about each (unless there's significant overlap between the two samples).

Let's say we have a hernia (ouch!) in the disease sample. This implies a hernia repair, but we may not have sampled that in the procedures for this patient. Then we have 12 stitches on the left arm in the procedures sample, implying a lacerated arm—but we may not have sampled that in the diseases for this patient. As shown in Table 6-2, a sample of only one value in each of two fields resulted in four pieces of background information, instead of two.

Table 6-2. A power of 1 means one disease, one procedure (bold = sampled)

Disease	Procedure	Background info
Hernia	Hernia repair	Hernia ⇒ Hernia repair
Lacerated arm	**12 stitches on left arm**	Lacerated arm ⇐ 12 stitches on left arm

Record sample

OK, so a random sample of each quasi-identifier might result in us assuming that the adversary has more background information than was intended, due to the strong correlation of health data across records. The obvious solution is therefore to sample by record! That way a hernia and its repair are in the same basket of information about the patient (Table 6-3). But isn't that cheating, because we now have less background information since one implies the other? Well, that's true only for strongly correlated information.

Sampling by record captures the connections between quasi-identifiers without us having to do it ourselves. Also, it's not likely for one piece of information in a quasi-identifier to imply all the others in the record. The lacerated arm could have been stitched up in an ambulance, an emergency room, or even a walk-in clinic. And odd pairings of disease and procedure will still stand out.

Table 6-3. Ah, this time we sample the record to get one disease, one procedure.

Disease	Procedure	Background info
Hernia	**Hernia repair**	Hernia, Hernia repair
Lacerated arm	12 stitches on left arm	(Not sampled)

Sample by visit

Another option is to sample by visit, so that we get a random sample of each quasi-identifier limited to a visit. This gives us a random sample, and the correlation of health information is in the sample so that it doesn't unintentionally inflate power. But in this case it's the correlation within a visit rather than a record. This approach is a bit more complicated, though, because we need to consider the diversity of the visits themselves, how many visits to sample, and how much information to sample per visit.

When sampling by visit, we also need a way to identify visits. Some data sets will have a visit identifier, so that we can track a visit over several days, but some data sets won't have this info. This isn't our preferred approach to sampling quasi-identifiers because it raises more questions than answers, especially when dealing with a wide range of data sets from different sources.

We prefer to sample by record. And once we have our sample of a patient's quasi-identifier values, we treat it as a basket of information for matching against all patients in a data set. The way the information was gathered is lost. We don't care about order, or visits, or claims. We just care about the information in the basket. In other words, we're assuming the adversary doesn't know how all the information is joined together.

Now, if we want two pieces of information from different quasi-identifiers to be connected, so that what happens to one also applies to the other, we define them as connected quasi-identifiers so that they aren't treated as two independent sources of information. We saw this concept in "Connected Variables" on page 64, and we'll see an example of it in the WTC disaster registry (it's easier to explain using an example).

The WTC Disaster Registry

Over 50,000 people are estimated to have helped with the rescue and recovery efforts after 9/11, and the medical records of over 27,000 of those are captured in the WTC disaster registry created by the Clinical Center of Excellence at Mount Sinai. Working with a variety of organizations, they reached out to recruit 9/11 workers and volunteers. Everyone who has participated in the registry has gone through a comprehensive series of examinations.[5] These include:

- Medical questionnaires
- Mental-health questionnaires
- Exposure assessment questionnaires
- Standardized physical examinations
- Optional follow-up assessments every 12 to 18 months

Capturing Events

We needed to convert the questionnaires and exams into a longitudinal data set we could work with—our methods don't apply directly to questionnaire data. So we needed to convert questions and exams into data we could process, then map the generalizations and suppression back to the questionnaires and exams. The registry is comprehensive and includes a lot of historical information gathered from patients. Unlike claims data, the WTC data contains no disease or procedure codes, no places of service (besides Mount Sinai), and no rows of information that organize the data set.

Instead, the registry presents a collection of health events, including information about when a specific health-related item is not a problem. That's something you don't see in claims data, unless there's a charge for that health-related item. Imagine an insurer charging you for not having a disease, or charging you for still having a disease even though you're not getting treatment for it! But since this kind of data is in the registry, and could be known to an adversary, we counted these as events.

After 9/11, the workers and volunteers became well known in their communities for their heroic efforts. This makes the information about them more prevalent, so we decided to connect the events to their respective dates. The visit date was used for questions that were specific to the date at which the visit occurred.

Thus, "Do you currently smoke?" would create an event for smoking at the time of visit, and "Have you been diagnosed with this disease?" would create an event for "no diagnosis" at the time of visit if the patient answered "no" to the question. Some questions included dates that could be used directly with the quasi-identifier and were more informative than the visit date. For example, the answer to "When were you diagnosed with this disease?" was used to provide a date for the disease event.

Ten years after the fact, however, it seems unlikely that an adversary will know the dates of a patient's events before 9/11. Often patients gave different years of diagnosis on follow-up visits because they themselves didn't remember what medical conditions they had! So instead of the date of event, we used "pre-9/11" as a value. But we made a distinction between childhood (under 18) and adulthood (18 and over) diagnoses, because this seemed like something an adversary could reasonably know.

These generalizations were done only for measuring risk, and weren't applied to the de-identified registry data. If the date can't be known to the adversary, there's no point in removing it from the original data. But before we get lambasted for this assumption, don't think that we left all those dates in their exact form in the data! We masked all dates to the same level of generalization that we used for the other events in the data, which we'll get to in the risk assessment.

The WTC Data Set

We'll start with the level 1 demographic data, because this is the data we assume to be known to an adversary (i.e., we don't use adversary power on level 1 data). The level 1 data in the registry already included generalizations used in the analyses conducted by Mount Sinai researchers. For example, date of birth was recorded for each patient, but the data set we received also included 5- and 10-year age groups. These generalizations were included because it's what researchers at Mount Sinai were using in their work.

We took the most general levels of the level 1 data available right off the bat. We did this because we knew, given all the background information about patients, that the risk of re-identification would be high. The only generalization we added was to divide height into four possible groups (<10th percentile, 10th to <50th percentile, 50th to <90th percentile, 90th percentile and higher).

Of course, if the risk had been well below our threshold, with minimal amounts of suppression, we would have gone back to try less general pieces of information (this didn't happen). But this seemed like a good starting point, since the level 1 data was already generalized to levels that were acceptable in the research being done at Mount Sinai.

The specific generalizations that were in the data aren't important, but the final level 1 data in Table 6-4 certainly is. This is because we include all level 1 data as part of what we assume an adversary knows, and because the more specific the demographic information is, the more identifiable a patient becomes.

Table 6-4. Level 1 quasi-identifiers

Field	Description
Gender	Patient's gender
Age	Patient's age (10-year groups)
Height	Patient's height (4 groups)
Language	Patient's native language (4 categories)
Race	Patient's race (6 categories)

The registry included a lot of information about patients, so we can give you only a taste of the level 2 event data in Table 6-5. We divided the events into three categories (based on the structure of the questionnaires and data): variable demographics, diseases (including mental health), and WTC exposures and activities.

Table 6-5. A sample of the possible events

Category of event	Event
Variable demographic	Job loss
Variable demographic	Separated or divorced
Variable demographic	Started or stopped smoking
Disease	Diagnosed with acute bronchitis
Disease	Diagnosed with sleep apnea
Disease	Diagnosed with panic disorder
WTC exposure or activity	Heavy equipment operator during 2011-09
WTC exposure or activity	Removal of debris during 2011-10
WTC exposure or activity	Supervisor of hazardous materials during 2011-10

The Power of Events

We specified a power level for each series of events. We chose a total power of 15 for longitudinal event data: a power of 5 for variable demographics, a power of 5 for disease events, and a power of 5 for mental health events. This means we assumed that an adversary would know up to 15 events about each individual in the registry.

The variability of patient events is at its maximum under this setup (i.e., $v = 1$), because we didn't include periods during which there was no change in a patient's quasi-identifiers, and we did include the year of the event in our analysis. If a patient was married in 2002 and divorced in 2006, we included this information as two events: 2002 married, and 2006 divorced. The patient's marital status could either be inferred or is missing for all other years, and therefore provides no further information. But there's no set of events (married, married, married), so variability is never "low."

Because we now have three main areas of patient information—variable demographics, diseases (including mental health), and 9/11 exposures—we assume a max adversary power of 15. Don't forget that we always include a patient's level 1 fixed demographics.

Adversary power applies to the longitudinal data only. This isn't a book of equations, but it's interesting (we think!) to see how our equation for adversary power works in this application. We have determined that p_{max} is 15, so we plug in $(p_{max} - 1) = 14$, and take out v because a divisor of 1 has no effect on the equation:

Adversary power (applied to WTC patient events)

$$p = \lceil 1 + 14 \times n \, / \, \max_{patients}(n) \rceil$$

Actually, there's a detail we skipped over. It's possible that patients with an abnormally high number of events could skew the equation. So, to get rid of outliers, we take the max to be the mean number of events per patient plus two standard deviations. For the WTC registry the mean number of events per patient was 103.8 (the median was 98), with a standard deviation of 52.7. This gives us a "max" of 209.2 events (the real max was 260, which just goes to show how much it can be skewed by an outlier):

Adversary power (applied to WTC patient events, no outliers)

$$p = \lceil 1 + 14 \times n \, / \, 209.2 \rceil$$

Given that the median number of events per patient was 98, half the patients had an adversary power of 1 to 8, and half had an adversary power of 9 to 15. That works out quite well. So, the more visits they attended, the higher the adversary power. This is exactly the way we want adversary power to work. The distribution of events in Figure 6-1 clearly shows the five visits in the data we looked at, and adversary power works out to be:

- 3–4 for one visit
- 7–8 for two visits
- 11–12 for three visits
- 14–15 for four visits
- 15 for five or more visits (power is at its maximum at this point)

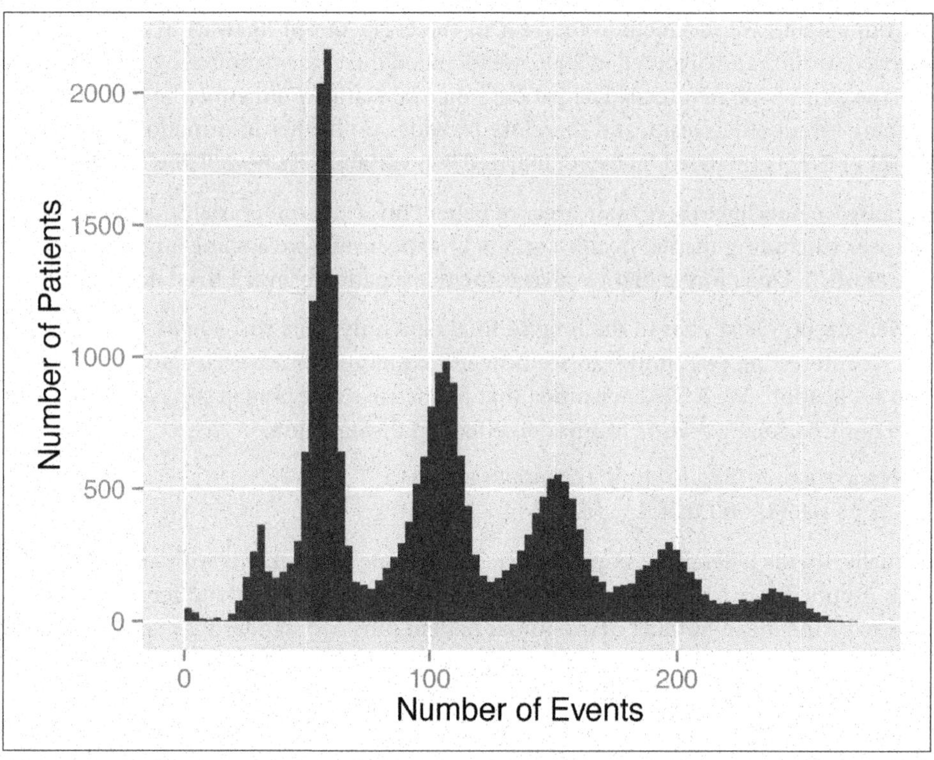

Figure 6-1. A roller coaster of events! The peaks represent the five visits, which show fewer and fewer patients attending follow-ups.

This change in power makes intuitive sense and captures the increase in background knowledge that an adversary would have as the number of patient visits rises. But the increase in adversary knowledge also affects fewer patients.

Risk Assessment

Now we're back to applying our methodology from Chapter 2. First and foremost, agreements were in place to limit the distribution of the data to a group of analysts, and these agreements prohibited the re-identification of individuals in the registry. The agreements also stipulated that if anyone in the registry were inadvertently identified, that information could not be disclosed to anyone. Period. Full stop.

Originally, Mount Sinai wanted the data to be treated as a public data release, which would warrant an overall risk threshold of 0.1. But the data was not being made public, and there were strong agreements in place, so we decided that an average risk of 0.15 would be appropriate.

Threat Modeling

Let's take a look at our three threats for this data set:

1. Because motives and capacity are low, but the extent of mitigating controls is also low, *Pr*(attempt) = 0.4. Basically, there are two ways that a re-identification attack might be launched: either through a deliberate attempt by the analyst, which is pretty unlikely given the explicit prohibition in the agreements, or through poor control over how data is handled, making it possible for someone on-site to attempt to re-identify the data. We assumed that the data users would only have to meet the HIPAA Security Rule requirements (see "Implementing the HIPAA Security Rule" on page 32 for more details on these).
2. You would probably be aware of it if someone you knew was a WTC first responder, since they did something truly awesome, and therefore so would an adversary. And given all the publicity and outreach involved in recruiting people, it's fair to assume that an adversary knows whether that person is also in the WTC registry. The probability of knowing a person in New York City who is in the WTC registry of 27,000 patients is *Pr*(acquaintance) = 0.39.
3. *Pr*(breach) = 0.27, based on our good old (for this book) historical data.

Results

Using adversary power, we were able to get the average risk below our threshold of 0.15 with some generalization and suppression, but nothing too crazy. We had to use the most generalized form of the level 1 data that was already provided by Mount Sinai, and we generalized dates to years (except the start dates of WTC efforts and service hours). Now, that might seem like a lot of generalization for dates, but keep in mind we're talking about either historical diagnoses, or the five visits (baseline plus follow-up). So, it's good enough for the analyses being considered.

There was also some suppression, but overall it worked out to be only 1% of the cells in the questionnaires. Now, because the level 1 data is always assumed to be known, it's almost always the case that this is the data that gets the most generalization and suppression. But this is way better than what would be achieved without power. In fact, we doubt that meaningful data can be disclosed at all without considering adversary power during the de-identification.

Final Thoughts

Adversary power is a great way to scale back our assumptions on longitudinal data from the "all-knowing" to the "some-knowing" adversary. Sampling the longitudinal data and scaling it based on the number and variability of the data is an extremely useful way to measure average risk. Keep in mind, though, that we don't apply these techniques blindly. If we know the data is out there somewhere, say publicly, and there's a risk that a data set will be matched to other data sets, then of course we need to go back a step and assume some form of omniscient adversary.

But in many cases, where there are controls on data (which is the case for many commercial data sets), this is the way to go. It allows us to decrease the amount of generalization and suppression needed to produce data sets that are useful for analytics. So it's a staple in our tool belt; you could say it's our power tool (ouch, bad pun!).

References

1. World Trade Center Medical Monitoring & Treatment Program (*http://bit.ly/wtc-program*)

2. M. Terrovitis, N. Mamoulis, and P. Kalnis, "Privacy-Preserving Anonymization of Set-Valued Data," Proc. *Very Large Databases Conference* (VLDB Endowment, 2008).

3. A. Maggurran, *Measuring Biological Diversity* (Hoboken, NJ: Wiley-Blackwell, 2004).

4. K. El Emam, L. Arbuckle, G. Koru, B. Eze, L. Gaudette, E. Neri, S. Rose, J. Howard, and J. Gluck, "De-identification Methods for Open Health Data: The Case of the Heritage Health Prize Claims Dataset," *Journal of Medical Internet Research* 14:1 (2012): e33.

5. J.M. Moline, R. Herbert, S. Levin, D. Stein, B.J. Luft, I.G. Udasin, and P.J. Landrigan, "WTC Medical Monitoring and Treatment Program: Comprehensive Health Care Response in Aftermath of Disaster," *Mount Sinai Journal of Medicine* 75:(2008): 67–75.

CHAPTER 7

Data Reduction: Research Registry Revisited

We often see massive data sets that need to be de-identified. With such large data sets, we are looking for ways to speed up the computations. We noted earlier that the de-identification process is often iterative, and it's important to expedite these iterations so we can reach a final data set rapidly. In enterprise settings there may be a time window for de-identification to complete so that subsequent analytics can be performed. This also demands more rapid execution of de-identification.

For large and complex data sets traditional de-identification may also result in considerable information loss. We therefore need to find ways to reduce the size and complexity of the data that minimize information loss but still provide the same privacy assurances.

The Subsampling Limbo

A straightforward data reduction approach is *subsampling*, in which we randomly sample patients from the data set to create a subset of records—the subset is the data set that is then released. The *sampling fraction* is the proportion of patients that are included in the subset. In the case of a cross-sectional data set, we sample based on records; in the case of a longitudinal data set, we sample based on patients instead. Otherwise, we could end up with a lot of records from those patients with an extreme number of records, even though they're in the minority. That wouldn't result in the correct sampling fraction, since we wouldn't have a representative subsample of patients. What we want is a data set that is representative of the whole.

This seems simple enough, and subsampling can actually be a very powerful way to reduce the re-identification risk. That's why national statistical agencies will generally only release a small subsample of census data—they do it as a way to manage re-identification risk. You may know that your neighbor A. Herring is in the census, because pretty much everyone is, but if the data being made publicly available is a random sample, then you don't know if A. Herring is included in the public data set or not.

How Low Can We Go?

Let's be clear, though: not all data users will be happy with a sample. Generally, data analysts want as much data as they can get. But apart from the general desire for more data, subsampling can also reduce the statistical power of many tests (just to be clear, this has nothing to do with adversary power, discussed in Chapter 6). So, subsampling won't always be the best option for reducing re-identification risk.

Our cutoff is a sample of 3,000—if a subsample is smaller than that, then the statistical power of classical tests will take a nontrivial hit.[1] But for samples of more than 3,000, the statistical power will be above 90% for most tests. When a data set might contain outliers or effects that are evident only in small groups, then 3,000 may be a low number even if the statistical power is high.

On the flip side, it's also possible to have too much data, resulting in models that are overfit and unreliable (i.e., they won't validate on external data). Studies have suggested a max of 20 effective observations per candidate predictor, but more for narrowly distributed predictors.[2] Things get more complicated for some models,[3] so really a power analysis involving effect size should be used to determine an appropriate sample size. And if this doesn't make any sense to you, then leave it to a statistician to sort out (they're good that way).

Not for All Types of Risk

For average risk, subsampling has a significant impact and can be another technique to use in addition to generalization and suppression. If a data user wants more precision on a variable (i.e., less generalization and suppression), then we can offer to use a smaller sampling fraction in order to bring the risk down.

But for maximum risk, the reality is that subsampling has very little impact. We would have to create a subsample that is extremely small for it to really have a meaningful impact on maximum risk. This means that for the public release of data sets, subsampling will not be a very useful technique to use (although it may still be worth doing, depending on the context and the changes in risk that you're looking for). However, for average risk it can have a nontrivial impact and is a useful technique to employ.

Remember that the subsampling we're talking about would be done completely at random, so it wouldn't bias the results of the analysis, and wouldn't require any special analytical methods. Of course, the subsampling can be done in a more complex way, where specific groups of observations are sampled less or more than others, but this also introduces complexities in risk measurement. And, to be honest, it would stretch the assumptions of current risk metrics and their estimators.

BORN to Limbo!

Let's use the BORN data, which we first saw in Chapter 3, to see how subsampling affects risk. We're disclosing the data to our good friend Researcher Ronnie, who now wants more precision in the variables and is willing to take a subsample to get it. The risk needs to be smaller than 0.115, and it's average risk since it's for a researcher. We use the same setup and quasi-identifiers as before, which we repeat in Table 7-1.

Table 7-1. Quasi-identifiers requested by Researcher Ronnie

Field	Description
BSex	Baby's sex
MDOB	Maternal date of birth
BDOB	Baby's date of birth
MPC	Maternal postal code

To give you a sense of things, we created random subsamples going down to only 5% of the data (OK, admittedly that's not much), and for each subsample we measured the average re-identification risk. This process was repeated 1,000 times and the mean risk across all iterations was computed. We compared the original data set to a version with generalization (but less than before), as described in Table 7-2, to see how we can change the precision of variables when we're subsampling.

Table 7-2. BORN again! Two versions of the data to see what subsampling will do to risk.

Data set	BSex	MDOB	BDOB	MPC
Original	No change	dd/mm/year	dd/mm/year	6 characters
With generalization	No change	year	week/year	3 characters

Now for the subsampling. Figure 7-1 shows that the average risk decreases rapidly as smaller samples are drawn. The question is, how low can we go? This is a dance we can only do with Researcher Ronnie, as he's the one that needs to work with the final subsampled data set.

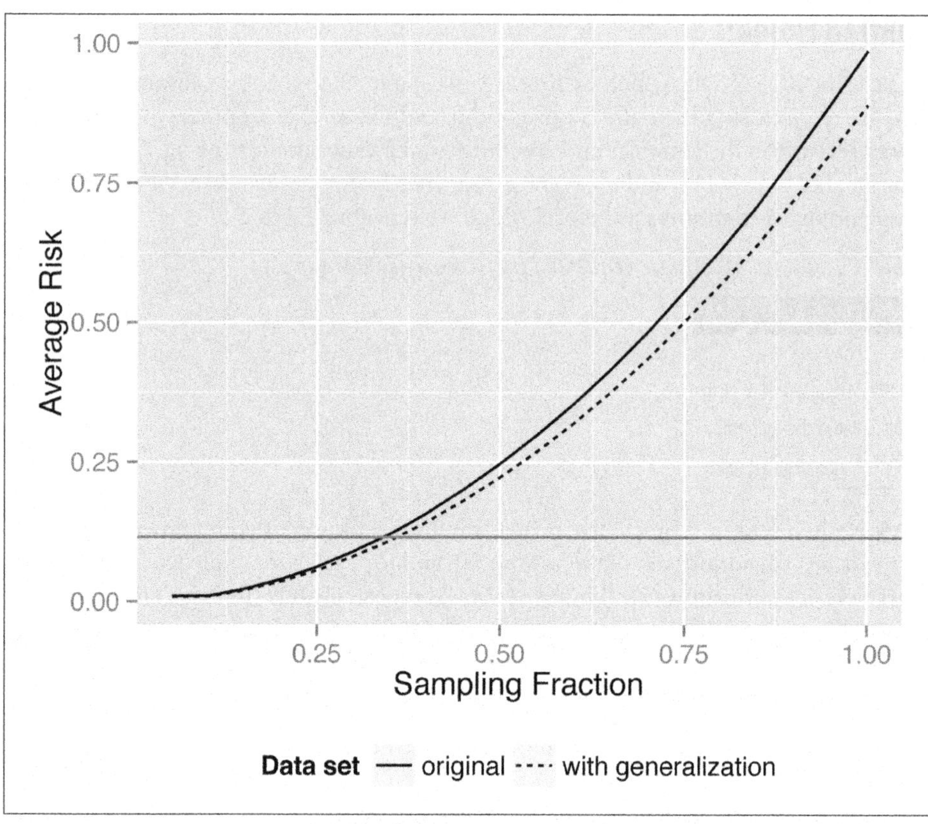

Figure 7-1. The lower Researcher Ronnie can go, the lower the risk

With all of the detailed variables and no generalization or suppression, subsampling achieves the 0.115 threshold with a sampling fraction of 0.3. The data set has 919,710 records, so a 30% subsample gives us 275,913 records. With generalization of the quasi-identifiers, we meet the risk threshold with a 35% subsample of 321,898 records. But the cost is a loss in precision on some of the quasi-identifiers.

If Researcher Ronnie wanted to perform detailed geospatial analysis, then he'd most likely want six-digit postal codes. With generalization on some of the other fields and suppression, we could even give him a larger subsample. It really comes down to what Researcher Ronnie needs, and how low he can go (in terms of sampling fraction, of course).

Many Quasi-Identifiers

Many health data sets have a large number of quasi-identifiers. We see that with registries and with survey data. A large number of variables might be collected directly from patients and their providers, or data might be linked with other data sets to create a much larger and more comprehensive data set. More quasi-identifiers means more opportunity to re-identify patients.

When there are a large number of quasi-identifiers, it is called "the curse of dimensionality." This means that there are too many variables, and the risk of re-identification is going to be quite large. To manage the risk in such cases using traditional assumptions and methods would result in excessive generalization and suppression. The data would have quite a lot of information removed from it.

But we have to be realistic with what we assume an adversary can know about patients. When there are a large number of quasi-identifiers, we don't have to consider all of them at the same time. If a data set has 20 quasi-identifiers, it's not reasonable to assume that an adversary would have 20 different pieces of background knowledge on any individual in the database. This is a lot of information about individuals, especially when we're referring to their physical or mental health. An adversary might only have five or seven pieces of background information that can be used for a re-identification attack.

This is the same concept of "adversary power" that we discussed in the context of the WTC registry, except now we are looking at adversary power from the perspective of a cross-sectional data set rather than a series of longitudinal events. The way we approach adversary power is a little different here because all of the patients will have the same number of quasi-identifiers (as opposed to each patient potentially having a different number of events), and we do not model diversity as that concept is not really applicable here.

If the 20 quasi-identifiers are strongly correlated, then knowing one quasi-identifier might be enough to estimate a few more. Bootstrapping this idea further, the adversary might only need to know three or five things to estimate the full set of 20 quasi-identifiers. But that doesn't change our approach, because evaluating the risk on a few quasi-identifiers would therefore be the same as looking at all the quasi-identifiers. So let's assume they're independent of one another.

Subsets of Quasi-Identifiers

Let's assume that the adversary could only reasonably know 5 of the 20 quasi-identifiers. The question then is which 5 out of 20 do we consider when evaluating the re-identification probability? We need to choose a subset of 5 fields to measure re-identification risk and to de-identify exposed records. Since any combination of 5 fields is plausible, this becomes a combinatorial problem—there are 15,504 combinations of 5 items from a set of 20 (better known as 20 choose 5, or, of 20 items, how many combinations of 5 can we choose?).

We could use a brute force approach and measure the re-identification risk for all 15,504 possible combinations of five quasi-identifiers. If the measured risk were high for any of these 15,504 combinations, then we would apply our de-identification algorithms. The problem is that evaluating 15,504 combinations can take a long time. And this solution doesn't scale well. For 21 fields, there are 20,249 combinations of 5; for 22 fields, there are 26,334 combinations; and so on. This would be a very inefficient way of solving the problem.

Let's consider some shortcuts. We'll refer to our quasi-identifiers as q_1 to q_{20}. We can consider each quasi-identifier individually; if the measured risk is high on any one individual quasi-identifier (say, q_1) then it will by definition be high for all combinations of five quasi-identifiers that include q_1. Date of birth is a good example, as it can be quite identifying. Grouped with state, gender, race, and body mass index, the main driver of risk would still be date of birth. The risk might be higher as a combination of five, but if it was already too high with date of birth then there's no need to evaluate the combination of quasi-identifiers.

On the other hand, even if the measured risk on q_1 is low, there may well be a combination of five quasi-identifiers that includes q_1 that has a high measured risk. Take age generalized into 10-year bands. That seems much less identifying, but pair it with state, gender, race, and body mass index, and suddenly we're not so sure. In this case we need to evaluate all combinations of five quasi-identifiers to ensure they have a low risk of re-identification. This isn't much of a shortcut, then, because we still need to check the combinations of five for many quasi-identifiers.

Another shortcut, which is more efficient but incurs a slight cost in terms of information loss, is to use covering designs. We can fine tune how much information loss is acceptable, balancing between precision and computation time.

Covering Designs

The idea of covering designs is to "cover" the combinations we're interested in with a larger group of combinations. It's easier to illustrate this with a small example. Let's say that we have five quasi-identifiers and we want to evaluate the risk of re-identification for all combinations of three quasi-identifiers. But we also want to minimize the number of combinations that we evaluate. Table 7-3 shows all combinations of 3 from 5. This gives us 10 combinations.

Table 7-3. Every combination of five quasi-identifiers taken three at a time

Set #	Combination
1	$\{q_1, q_2, q_3\}$
2	$\{q_1, q_2, q_4\}$
3	$\{q_1, q_2, q_5\}$
4	$\{q_1, q_3, q_4\}$
5	$\{q_1, q_3, q_5\}$

Set #	Combination
6	$\{q_1, q_4, q_5\}$
7	$\{q_2, q_3, q_4\}$
8	$\{q_2, q_3, q_5\}$
9	$\{q_2, q_4, q_5\}$
10	$\{q_3, q_4, q_5\}$

Now let's consider the fewest possible blocks of size 4, or combinations of four quasi-identifiers, that cover all combinations of three quasi-identifiers. This is shown in Table 7-4. Here we managed to reduce the number of combinations from 10 to 4, but we still evaluate all possible combinations of three quasi-identifiers from a set of five. Table 7-4 is a (5,4,3) covering design (like 5 choose 3, except we add a middle piece, which is the block size, so that it's more like 5 choose blocks of 4 to cover combinations of 3).

Table 7-4. Covering every combination of five quasi-identifiers taken three at a time in blocks of four

Block	Set #'s covered
$\{q_1, q_2, q_3, q_4\}$	1, 2, 4, 7
$\{q_1, q_2, q_3, q_5\}$	1, 3, 5, 8
$\{q_1, q_2, q_4, q_5\}$	2, 3, 6, 9
$\{q_1, q_3, q_4, q_5\}$	4, 5, 6, 10

When we measure the re-identification probability for a covering design, we take the maximum probability across the combinations that are evaluated and use that as the measure for the whole data set. The rotten apple spoils the barrel. We've developed a strategy to minimize the amount of information loss. Compared to other strategies we tried, this one has resulted in the least distortion of the data:

1. Sort the blocks in the covering design by the percent of records that are high risk, with the largest percentages on top.
2. Starting from the top, apply generalization followed by suppression to the block until the risk is acceptably low.
3. Continue down the list of blocks, using generalization and suppression, until the risk is acceptably low for all of them.

Starting from the top of the list of blocks, applying generalization and suppression lowers the risk for the other blocks lower down the list as well. In a lot of cases that means we don't need to do anything to the blocks lower down the list, since the worst was dealt with first.

Covering BORN

We linked the BORN data set to socioeconomic data from the census, available at the postal code level. The census provides aggregate numbers, not exact matches to the individual records in BORN. There might be 30 people in postal code P0M1B0 that are visible minorities, but we don't know which, if any, of these are in the BORN data. The only option to get the exact numbers would be to use secure linking, which we'll discuss in Chapter 12. The other way is to simulate it. If we know there are 200 people in P0M1B0, then we randomly assign the status of visible minority to individual records with that same postal code, with a probability of 15% (30/200). For our purposes, we used the simulation approach to assign a value to each record in the BORN registry.

Linking BORN, with five quasi-identifiers, to the census data added seven quasi-identifiers to the maternal-health registry (see Table 7-5). Using covering designs makes the de-identification of this data set a lot faster. Compared to a brute force approach of evaluating all combinations, many fewer combinations of quasi-identifiers need to be evaluated.

Table 7-5. BORN and census quasi-identifiers

Origin	Variable	Description
BORN	BSex	Baby's sex
BORN	MDOB	Maternal date of birth
BORN	BDOB	Baby's date of birth
BORN	MPC	Maternal postal code
BORN	PBabies	Number of previous live births
BORN	LHIN	The health region where the birth occurred
BORN	LANGUAGE	Language spoken at home (this field also appears in the census)
BORN	ABORIGN	Aboriginal status
BORN	MINORITY	Visible minority
Census	MSTATUS	Marital status
Census	IMMIGRATION	Immigration status
Census	OCCUPATION	Occupation category
Census	PGROUP	Population group (e.g., West Indian, East Asian, Arab, African, and so on)
Census	INCOME	Income in $10k increments
Census	CERT	Highest educational certificate obtained

In general, the number of blocks goes down as the block size increases (as you would expect). This can really speed up computations. However, the larger the blocks are, the more we end up overestimating the actual probability of re-identification, which results in more distortion to the data than is strictly necessary. We show this in Table 7-6, which is independent of the data. Note that the first entry for a covering, (15,*k*,*k*), is equivalent to all combinations (15 choose *k*), the worst case.

Table 7-6. A cover up, to reduce the number of quasi-identifiers we need to consider. The numbers in this table are the numbers of blocks we need to evaluate.

Block size (k)	(15,*k*,3)	(15,*k*,5)	(15,*k*,7)
3	455		
4	124		
5	56	3003	
6	31	578	
7	15	189	6435
8	13	89	871
9	10	42	270
10	7	27	108

Final Thoughts

If you're using average risk, subsampling is a simple and very effective way to lower the potential for re-identification. Not so much for maximum risk. Just make sure you have some idea of what kind of analytics will be performed, and you can probably limbo to a pretty low subsample and not have to worry. A power analysis would be a great way to be sure. In another dimension, you could have too many quasi-identifiers, and covering designs can help manage the risk in a more reasonable way than assuming the adversary knows all of them. All in all, it's just more tools to help manage risk and our assumptions.

References

1. J. Cohen, *Statistical Power Analysis for the Behavioral Sciences*, 2nd ed. (Hillsdale, NJ: LEA Publishers, 1988).

2. F.E. Harrell Jr., *Regression Modeling Strategies: With Applications to Linear Models, Logistic Regression, and Survival Analysis* (New York: Springer, 2001).

3. T. Snijders and R. Bosker, *Multilevel Analysis: An Introduction to Basic and Advanced Multilevel Modeling* (London: SAGE Publications, 1999).

CHAPTER 8

Free-Form Text: Electronic Medical Records

It might seem like a somewhat trivial task to find and anonymize all personal health information in a document, and there's research in the academic literature about this, but here we're interested in where the rubber meets the road. It's not enough for a system to catch 80% of the names in a medical document—it has to catch *all* of them or it's considered a breach. That means our standards have to be much higher than what you'd typically find.

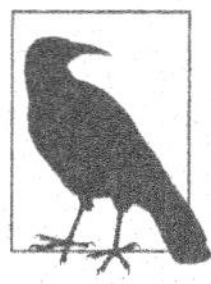

You'll notice that we're dealing with both direct and indirect identifiers when processing free-form text. Both types of identifiers are extracted from the text and dealt with in the same way (e.g., tagging or redaction). So does that make text de-identification a form of masking or a form of de-identification, as we've defined them earlier in this book? In fact, it's both. That's why we call it text *anonymization.*

Not So Regular Expressions

Many modern clinical systems have free-form text: nurses' notes, consultation letters, radiology reports, pathology reports, and so on. This text gets into electronic systems through health care providers who input the data. Even though electronic medical records allow the entry of structured information, sometimes using these systems takes longer than just writing in the information (for example, choosing a diagnosis from a long drop-down list), and if no analytics will be performed on this data that will directly inform their practice (which is commonly the case), there is no incentive to take the time to enter structured data. So we end up with a lot of free-form text.

This text is a very rich source of information for analytics purposes. But before we can pass such data through an analytics pipeline it needs to be anonymized, as is the case for structured data.

Text found in clinical systems is different from what you'd find from other sources (for example, in newspaper articles or research articles). For one thing, most of it is never edited, which means a lot of typos, shorthand, incomplete sentences, spelling errors, and poor grammar. The text might even come from automated transcription of a dictation, or be the output of optical character recognition software transferring handwritten notes. Sometimes these methods may work out great, but other times they may perform poorly. Remember that many facilities have legacy systems and hardware, and that there are still many old and less than perfect tools in use today.

Still, what we call free-form text data will have some structure in a health care setting. For example, an extract from an electronic medical record may have the name of the patient at the top, as part of a header, with the patient's medical record number, the date of the visit, and the name of the physician writing the note. These four fields would be the structured component of the text data. After those fields would come the true free-form text component, consisting of the notes from medical staff.

Another example of somewhat structured free-form text data is an XML file with predefined elements and attributes. An XML document may be exported from an electronic medical record system or be part of a feed from a medical device. Some of these XML documents may specifically tag the name of the patient, but some may be comments or notes as free-form text. It really depends on the context, and the variety of text formats themselves can add to the challenge of anonymization.

When there's some predefined structure to a data set, we can take advantage of it during the anonymization. For example, if we know from the structured field that a patient's name is "David Greybeard," then whenever we encounter "David" or "Dave" in the free-form text portion we'll know that it's likely referring to that same patient.

When the free-form text data comes from a known system, such as an electronic medical record, we can also pull out the list of names of all patients and all physicians, and create a list of names and aliases that can be used as a lookup dictionary. These lists, for example, can be used as part of the anonymization since the vast majority of names in the data set will be of those patients and physicians.

But we want to give you a general presentation of text anonymization here, without getting bogged down in the wide variety of electronic medical record systems and how they are structured. So, we'll ignore the techniques we just mentioned that take advantage of structured information, and focus on the anonymization of the free-form text component itself.

General Approaches to Text Anonymization

There are two general approaches to solving this problem: model based, and heuristic or rule based (which we'll simply refer to as rule based, because it sounds a lot less complicated). A model-based approach derives a statistical or machine learning model from a training data set, then applies that model to new data. In a rule-based approach, the anonymization system applies a predefined set of criteria and constraints directly on the data set without the need for any training. (Well, not exactly—the training in this case came from researchers and analysts that figured out the rules. But we can take the rules themselves, once formulated, and just apply them directly to the free-form text data.) Another option is to combine the model-based and rule-based approaches into a hybrid system, to get the best of their strengths and, hopefully, lessen their weaknesses.

Anonymization tools could be deployed in a large institution, or in many small practices and clinics. By "large institution" we mean something like the veterans' administration or a teaching hospital. A large institution would be a good place for a model-based system because it would have the resources to create an annotated data set to be used for training the model. We've found that many small practices and clinics, though, don't seem to fit with the model-based approach. They just don't have the capacity or expertise to invest in training the model. And because of this, they often aren't willing to try using model-based systems. That poses some unique challenges, as rule-based systems may have limits in terms of what they can realistically do.

Training the model is really important because you need details from the local environment to calibrate its settings. Training a model on one institution's data and then using it on another institution's data will not work very well—the model will just not be that accurate. Also, the document types matter. Imagine a model that was trained by anonymizing the free-form text in pathology reports but was then applied to radiology reports. Again, the contexts are completely different. The shorthand used will vary; the medical terms will vary; even the structure of sentences may vary. Context matters to a model-based system. If a training data set isn't available, the only way a model will meet your needs is if it starts with a reasonable set of rules (yes, we're back to the hybrid system).

To get a model-based system to work to its full potential, though, we need a good local training data set. That means extracting a sample of historical data that is representative of the whole, and manually annotating it. Annotation is a time-consuming and labor-intensive exercise, and it's best done by someone with some medical training who can correctly recognize medical terms in the text. The amount of annotation will depend on the modeling technique, but we estimate that in general at least 100 documents need to be annotated manually to get the system up and running. But that's only a starting point. A much larger number of documents would need to be manually annotated to build a training data set that ensures the model is stable across document types.

Ideally, you'd have a team of people with medical training doing the manual annotation to build a really good training data set. They could work together, pooling resources and brainpower, with each person responsible for a specific set of documents. You'd probably also want one highly reliable senior person to perform manual annotation on a sample of each person's documents, to see how much they agree (there are statistical ways to do this). Or, if you have the resources, you could have people work on the same documents, and allow them to discuss discrepancies between their work and resolve differences. One highly reliable senior person would again be needed, this time to adjudicate on any unresolved differences.

However, we've found that many organizations, big and small, are unwilling to make the investment to produce good training sets. They don't want to be bothered with assigning medically trained staff to manually annotate documents, given all of their more pressing needs. What they want is a system that works immediately, no muss or fuss. So we'll instead focus on rule-based approaches. Do keep in mind, though, that model-based systems can have some performance advantages in detecting personal information in free-form text. What's more important in the context of our discussion are the metrics we'll discuss for evaluating these systems, rule or model based.

Ways to Mark the Text as Anonymized

The purpose of a text anonymization system is to extract personal information from text. There are different elements we want to extract. A list of some of the obvious direct and indirect identifiers is presented in Table 8-1. Once these elements are extracted, we can then anonymize them in a number of different ways: redaction by replacing them with some form of indicator, like "***"; tagging with their type; randomization within their type; and generalization into a less-specific type.

Table 8-1. Some identifiers we need to extract

Direct identifier	Indirect identifier
First and middle name	Age
Last name	Postal/ZIP code
Street	Date
Email	Health care facility
Phone number	City and state
ID	Country

Redaction is the simplest post-processing approach, but it's also the least informative. It's the classic spy movie style of removing secret information from documents by blacking it out. It shows that there was some personal information in that space, and that it was removed. But anyone looking at the data gets no indication of the type of information that was removed. Sometimes redaction is acceptable if the type of analysis that will be performed on the anonymized text does not need to use direct or indirect identifiers. For example, if the analysis is to classify the patient into one of a number of possible diagnoses or by severity of disease, whether he was "Dave" or "Al" will not really make a difference to that task.

Tagging at least replaces the element with the type of information that was removed. For example, "David" can be replaced by "<FIRST_NAME>." Because there could be multiple first names in the text, we can also index them. Every instance of "David" could be replaced with the tag "<FIRST_NAME:1>," and if there's another name in the text such as "Jane," good, all we need to do is replace this with another tag, "<FIRST_NAME: 2>." That way the reader of the anonymized text will know when the same person is being referred to repeatedly in another part of the same document.

Randomization is the same scheme that's used for dealing with direct identifiers in structured data. We simply replace every instance of "David" with a randomly selected name from a names database (for example, a names database obtained from the census). We can even be smart about it and replace "David" with a name that's typically associated with the same sex, in this case a male name, like "Flint." Generalization would also work the same way as with structured data, where a generalized value is used to replace the original value in the text.

Evaluation Is Key

The challenge with text anonymization is the detection itself. Finding elements of personal information in the text is not always straightforward. Text anonymization systems are obviously evaluated based on how well they can detect the various elements of personal information, but you need to evaluate how well a text anonymization system detects personal information to determine whether it's right for the job.

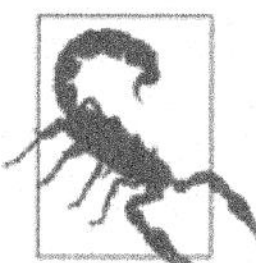

Strict but appropriate criteria help to guide modifications and improvements. If the evaluation is weak, personal information could be inadvertently leaked in the text that was supposed to be anonymized. If that text is then released, there's a good chance it will be considered a breach.

We call any record with free-form text a *document*. The collection of documents that form a large and structured set of texts is called a *corpus* (Latin for "body"). We want to evaluate the performance of a text anonymization system on the corpus (certainly not a *corpus vile*, or worthless body, for our purposes).

We want to be sure that elements of personal information are detected with high accuracy per document. Assume a document has 10 last names in it: if we detect and redact 9 of those last names but fail to detect even 1 of them, this is considered a disclosure. It doesn't matter that 90% of the last names were detected and redacted—that last name would result in the identification of an individual. The document would have to be considered to have personal information in it. This is considered an "all or nothing" approach to evaluation.

By way of comparison, consider a record in a structured data set. If there's enough information left behind after anonymization that David Greybeard can be associated to the record, the record can be re-identified. It doesn't matter that we protected most of David's record—the record is still re-identifiable. That's bad, and we wouldn't accept this for structured data. The same rules have to apply to free-form text.

In the text anonymization system with 1 leaked name out of 10, we had a 100% failure rate on that document, not a 90% success rate. This distinction is important because it can have a huge impact on how we measure the performance of the text anonymization system on a corpus. If we had a second document where 80% of the identifiers were detected and redacted, the overall performance of the system would not be an average of 85%, but 0%. Of course, if these were the only two documents out of 100 in which names had not been detected, then the average performance of the system would be 98%. The point here is that we're evaluating performance based on the number of documents that have leaks in the corpus, not the number of individual names themselves that are leaked.

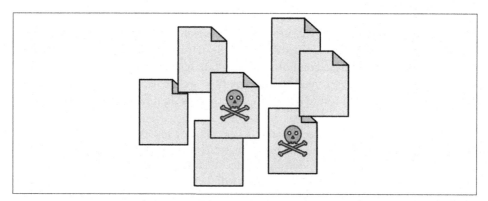

Figure 8-1. If even one identifier is leaked in a document, it's a disclosure. The two documents with leaks represent failures of the text anonymization system to detect personal information.

This is far stricter than the criteria typically used when evaluating text anonymization systems, but it's consistent with privacy regulations. Privacy regulations do not provide a "free pass" to free-form text. A data set needs to have a low risk of re-identification, irrespective of its format.

When we evaluate the performance of an anonymization system, we need to make a distinction between direct and indirect identifiers—they have a different standard for what's deemed "acceptable risk." For starters, if we're able to detect one type of personal information very well and another one poorly, if we pool their results we might lose this distinction between the two types of personal information. We need to know whether one element is detected poorly. For direct identifiers, the standards of acceptable detection on the corpus have to be very high—close to perfection—because, well, they're *directly* identifiable! We can't miss these. For indirect identifiers, however, we can be a bit more lax. In this case we can use standards similar to what we use for structured data.

Let's first examine the metrics to use before covering acceptable detection rates.

Appropriate Metrics, Strict but Fair

We'll use the confusion matrix in Table 8-2 to help illustrate how we define three metrics. If the text anonymization system tagged "chimpanzee" as a FIRST_NAME when it isn't one, that's a false positive (*FP*). If the system didn't detect "Jane" as a FIRST_NAME, that's a false negative (*FN*). An element that's correctly identified ("Greybeard" is a LAST_NAME) is a true positive (*TP*), and an element that's not personal information that was ignored ("banana") is a true negative (*TN*).

Table 8-2. A confusion matrix, just to confuse you (PI = personal information)

	Recognized element of PI	Unrecognized element of PI
Element of PI	True positive (*TP*)	False negative (*FN*)
Not element of PI	False positive (*FP*)	True negative (*TN*)

With those definitions in place, we can describe some metrics using that confusion matrix. As you can imagine, there could be a very large number of true negatives in a document. We don't want to include these in any metrics, as they would skew the evaluations. Of the elements that were recognized as personal information (the second column of the confusion matrix), we're interested in the proportion that were correctly recognized, known as the *precision*. This can also be interpreted as the probability of a recognized element actually being personal information:

Precision (or Positive Predictive Value)
: $Precision = TP \,/\, (TP + FP)$

We're also interested in the proportion of these elements of personal information that were correctly recognized, known as *recall*. Similar to precision, this can be interpreted as the probability that an element of personal information is recognized:

Recall (or Sensitivity or True Positive Rate)
: $Recall = TP \,/\, (TP + FN)$

We can summarize these two results into a single metric, known as the *F*-measure, using the harmonic mean of precision and recall. It's a form of balanced average appropriate for rates. Although this combined measure is an easy way to look at both precision and recall together, it's always better to consider all three metrics:

F-measure (or F-score)
: $F\text{-}measure = 2 \,/\, (\,(1 \,/\, Recall) + (1 \,/\, Precision)\,)$

In practice, we can also weight precision and recall differently, using a weighted harmonic mean. A low precision value means that the text anonymization system is redacting too much information that it doesn't need to. This reduces the utility of the anonymized data. A low recall value means that the system is not detecting elements of personal information and, depending on the threshold selected, could be considered a privacy breach. So we may prefer to use an alternative weighting. A popular choice is the F_2-measure, where recall is weighted higher than precision. This places more emphasis on avoiding the risk of leaving in elements of personal information:

F_2-measure

$$F_2\text{-}measure = 5 / ((4 / Recall) + (1 / Precision))$$

Text anonymization is, at heart, an information extraction task. These metrics have a long-standing tradition of use in the field of information retrieval,[1] and are also used in evaluating the detection of personal health information.[2, 3]

Standards for Recall, and a Risk-Based Approach

From a re-identification risk perspective, some experts in this area have set standards for recall (ensuring elements of personal information are in fact detected). In the case of direct identifiers, recall needs to be close to 95% or higher to be acceptable.[3] This would allow a minimal number of direct identifiers to be missed.

For indirect identifiers, we can apply a risk-based approach that fits nicely with our previously described methodology. We can say that an adversary would need to have at least two indirect identifiers—not detected in the same document—to re-identify someone. Two may seem like an arbitrary number, but if only one were needed it would likely be a direct identifier, not an indirect one. There's evidence that Canadians can be re-identified with a very high probability using only two indirect identifiers (date of birth and postal code)[4] and similar results have been seen in European countries. In the US, two pieces of information (date of birth and five-digit ZIP code) are believed to uniquely characterize approximately 63% of the population.[5]

Now we need to tie this in with our risk-based approach to anonymization. If we let r be the recall for indirect identifiers, the probability of two indirect identifiers being missed during anonymization is given by $Pr(\text{missed}) = (1 - r)^2$. So, anything greater than two indirect identifiers would actually be less conservative, which is why we limit ourselves to two. Let's revisit our four attacks from Chapter 2 and reframe them in the context of free-form text anonymization with indirect identifiers.

For example, we can consider attack T1, a deliberate attempt at re-identification, and define the overall risk of re-identification. But now we include the probability of missing an indirect identifier, because it really depends on whether or not the text anonymization system detects it in the first place. The risk here is that it doesn't detect an indirect identifier. If two indirect identifiers are missed in a document, then it's possible that a patient could be re-identified.

Attack T1 (Text)
: $Pr(\text{re-id} \mid \text{attempt, missed}) \times Pr(\text{attempt} \mid \text{missed}) \times Pr(\text{missed})$

So, for a re-identification to occur, the anonymization system needs to have missed at least two indirect identifiers. If that happens, an adversary must attempt to re-identify the data. And if that happens, we're interested in the probability of an individual being re-identified from these two pieces of information.

For the purpose of a simple example, let's say we want this overall probability to be less than or equal to 0.05, assuming we're treating it as a public data release:

Risk (Text)
: $Pr(\text{re-id} \mid \text{attempt, missed}) \times Pr(\text{attempt} \mid \text{missed}) \times (1 - r)^2 \leq 0.05$

If we assume that two indirect identifiers can re-identify someone with certainty, we can simplify the equation by letting $Pr(\text{re-id} \mid \text{attempt, missed}) = 1$. This is more or less true in the Canadian context, and a bit conservative in the US context (assuming date of birth and postal code or five-digit ZIP code).

For the BORN registry (introduced in Chapter 3), we determined that the probability of a re-identification attempt is 0.4. By rearranging the preceding risk equation, with $Pr(\text{attempt} \mid \text{missed}) = 0.4$, we find the acceptable recall for the anonymization of free-form text in this case is $r \geq 1 - \sqrt{(0.05/0.4)} = 0.65$. As this simple example demonstrates, with this risk-based scheme the appropriate recall is determined by context.

The same reasoning can be applied to the remaining attacks to set the appropriate recall threshold. The maximum recall across all relevant attacks is the recall value that will be used to anonymize the data (anything lower will not meet the recall threshold for at least one attack, i.e., the one with the max recall). But remember that the acceptable thresholds to use for direct and indirect identifiers are very different when deciding whether the anonymization system is defensible.

Standards for Precision

Deciding what's an acceptable minimum level of precision is more challenging because it's largely a reflection of data quality. Some experts in this area have suggested a precision of 80% for direct identifiers and 70% for indirect identifiers,[3] and we agree with these thresholds.

But unlike the "all-or-nothing" approach to calculating recall across documents, precision can be calculated as a "micro-average." A micro-average pools all of the elements that have been extracted as protected health information (PHI) by the anonymization system and calculates precision directly, ignoring whether the elements of PHI came from different documents. Basically we treat the corpus as one big document. So it's not precision per document, but precision across all documents. This makes sense because we're interested in whether or not the system recognized PHI correctly, and the distinction between documents doesn't matter in this case.

Anonymization Rules

There are a lot of things to consider when developing an anonymization system for free-form text.[6] We'll examine a few of the major ones.

First and foremost, keep in mind that there will be all kinds of errors in the text. This isn't a slight on doctors' handwriting, but a recognition of reality. Medical staff have to use tablets with virtual keyboards, or enter information at terminal stations while hurriedly trying to look after multiple patients, and so on and so forth. Lookup lists of names and the like are an important part of the process of detecting personal information, but all these errors will limit their usefulness. And where lookup lists are used, they need to include shorthand, nicknames, and any other variants you can think of.

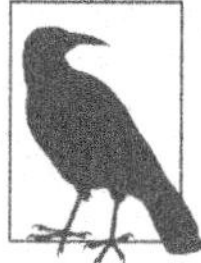

When looking up names, it's usually better to use a distance measure, or edit distance (in a broad sense), to capture words that are "close" to matching. That way some spelling errors will not completely trip up the system. The common edit distance is the Levenshtein distance, which basically measures the number of single-character edits required to get from one word to another.

There are a lot of examples of variants besides just typos and the like—there are also variants for drug and disease names. People often say aspirin, but the chemical name is acetylsalicylic acid (good luck trying to spell that under pressure), or ASA. Drugs can also be referred to by brand names (Advil) or generic names (ibuprofen), and they could have different names in different countries (acetaminophen in North America, or paracetamol in Europe). Shorthand can vary widely between departments, although there are some common ones, like hep B for hepatitis B, or HBV for the hep B virus, depending on the context.

Acronyms can be confused with common medical nomenclature. Confusion can also arise when dealing with postal codes: consider maternal pregnancy history depicted as G2P1A1 denoting gravida 2, parity 1, and abortions 1; C6C7T1 denoting cervical spine 6, cervical spine 7, and thoracic spine 1; or S1S2S4 nomenclature denoting heart sounds.

Names of people can also cause all sorts of confusion. They could clash with months of the year (April), and there are eponyms to worry about, where a person's name could be a disease (Huntington), an index (Apgar), or a procedure (Bankart). These are direct identifiers, so it's important to be able to distinguish between these examples and actual names, maybe using the context to figure it out. One way to do this is to have "exclusion lists" of procedure, index, and disease names that are not identified as people's names.

Similar problems exist with location names (no one said this would be easy). Fergus Falls is a city in Minnesota, and "Fergus falls" is the description of some guy taking a fall. What if they're not properly capitalized? Vienna, Wien, and Vena are all the capital of Austria (why it has three capitals is not clear). Villa Maria is the name of a villa, and it's an area in Montreal. The Big Apple is New York or someone's lunch, and the Pittsburgh of the South is the US city of Birmingham. All of these variants, composite names, and nicknames will add confusion to a text anonymization system.

Informatics for Integrating Biology and the Bedside (i2b2)

Informatics for Integrating Biology and the Bedside, better known as i2b2, is a research center in biomedical computing[7] that endeavors to be at the cutting edge of genomics and biomedical informatics. The center is comprised of six cores:

- (Core 1) Science
- (Core 2) Driving biology projects
- (Core 3) Infrastructure
- (Core 4) Education
- (Core 5) Dissemination
- (Core 6) Administration

It provides data other researchers can use in their own work, and in this case text data for anonymization. We'll use this text data to show how the methods we've presented can be used in practice, but of course the results carry over to other data sets.

i2b2 Text Data Set

i2b2 has made publicly available a set of 889 discharge records from various medical departments of the health care system in Boston, MA, USA. These documents were manually annotated by a group of people and all personal health identifiers were replaced with supposedly realistic surrogates. But it's far from perfect.

If you look at the names in the i2b2 documents closely you'll find <PHI TYPE="PATIENT">Flytheleungfyfe</PHI>, <PHI TYPE="PATIENT">Cornea</PHI>, <PHI TYPE="DOCTOR">ah / BMot </PHI>, and <PHI TYPE="DOCTOR">A HAS</PHI>. Or how about <PHI TYPE="DOCTOR">Ala Aixknoleskaysneighslemteelenortkote</PHI>, a last name with 35 letters? Those are some very strange names, and this weirdness happens for at least 10% of the tagged PHI (maybe even as high as 25%).

We use this data set because it's generally available, and it's been used in a number of other evaluative studies. This would make it useful for comparisons, except that most, if not all, other free-form text anonymization systems have been evaluated using much less strict metrics.

The odd names tagged as PHI also make this rule-based system seem to perform far worse than it really would, because it's very unlikely that any rules or lists will include these strange names. You can imagine that a model-based system might train on a lot of these oddities and therefore seem to perform better, but this might be very misleading. A rule-based system could be tuned to deal with such text, but that wouldn't be useful for real text. i2b2 records are what they are, but we changed some of the annotations to make them more realistic and produce more meaningful results.

We divided the documents into two parts: a training set of 589 documents (66% of the corpus) and a test set of 300 documents (34% of the corpus). Let's consider a few summary statistics to show you what the data is like (nothing fancy, just a frequency count, mean, median, standard deviation, and interquartile range of the number of identifiers per document). First we have the training documents, with summaries in Table 8-3.

Table 8-3. Per-element summary statistics of the i2b2 training subset of 589 documents (IQR = interquartile range)

PHI element	Count	Mean	Median	Std. dev.	IQR
First name	2237	3.79	4.00	2.17	3
Middle name	280	0.47	0.00	0.92	1
Last name	3257	5.52	5.00	3.74	4
Email	357	0.60	1.00	0.48	1
Date	5115	8.68	8.00	5.02	5
Phone number	133	0.22	0.00	0.56	0
Health care facility	1715	2.91	2.00	2.34	3
Age	12	0.02	0.00	0.14	0
ID	3118	5.29	5.00	1.32	2
Street	24	0.04	0.00	0.22	0
City	163	0.27	0.00	0.73	0
State	66	0.11	0.00	0.40	0
ZIP code	11	0.01	0.00	0.16	0

Then there are the testing documents, with summaries in Table 8-4. Overall they're very similar subsets of the corpus, but note that there's a lot of variation in the number of names and dates per document (although this shouldn't come as any surprise).

Table 8-4. Per-element summary statistics of the i2b2 training subset of 300 documents

PHI element	Count	Mean	Median	Std. dev.	IQR
First name	1092	3.64	4.00	1.44	1
Middle name	146	0.48	0.00	0.87	1
Last name	1411	4.70	4.00	2.26	3
Email	261	0.87	1.00	0.33	0
Date	1983	6.61	6.00	3.82	3
Phone number	99	0.33	0.00	0.54	1
Health care facility	685	2.28	2.00	1.43	2
Age	4	0.01	0.00	0.14	0
ID	1690	5.63	6.00	0.86	1
Street	10	0.03	0.00	0.19	0
City	50	0.16	0.00	0.66	0
State	31	0.10	0.00	0.44	0
ZIP code	5	0.01	0.00	0.12	0

Risk Assessment

Let's assume we're disclosing the i2b2 data set to Researcher Ronnie (him again!), who'll use it to develop machine learning models to classify patients based on their tendency to be readmitted. Given that the i2b2 data has been selected specifically for sharing, there are no sensitive diagnoses in there. So we'll use a threshold of 0.1 for the overall risk.

Threat Modeling

We need to consider the three attacks T1, T2, and T3 from "Step 3: Examining Plausible Attacks" on page 26:

1. If Researcher Ronnie follows the HIPAA Security Rule (described in "Implementing the HIPAA Security Rule" on page 32), *Pr*(attempt) = 0.4, giving us a minimum recall of $r \geq 1 - \sqrt{(0.1/0.4)} = 0.5$.
2. There were 845,806 discharges in the state in 2006,[8] which gives us a prevalence of 0.001 and a probability of knowing someone who has been discharged from a hospital of *Pr*(acquaintance) = 0.145. This gives us a minimal recall of 0.17 under attack T2.
3. For a data breach we already have *Pr*(breach) = 0.27, based on historical data, giving us a minimum recall of 0.39.

Based on these three attacks, we have to take the strictest minimum recall, which is the 0.5 found for T1. Using this minimum recall makes sure that the overall risk of re-identification for this data set is at or below 0.1. For precision, we used the threshold of 80% defined in "Standards for Precision" on page 121.

A Rule-Based System

We built a rule-based system to illustrate how anonymization works in practice, and also to set a baseline for the kind of performance that you can expect from such a system. The basic rule-based system that we developed has a total of 125 rules, summarized in Table 8-5. By "basic" we mean a dozen pages of rules, and you could write a textbook about how this was done, so we'll leave it at that.

Table 8-5. The number of rules by element type

PHI type	Number of rules
Person names (first, middle, last names)	36
Phone number	12
Date	20
Email	2
ID	18
Age	1
Organization	14
Location (street, city, state, country, ZIP code)	26

Results

We used the i2b2 documents in our rule-based system, using our strict metrics, to evaluate its ability to anonymize free-form text. The rules were constructed using the training documents, and were then evaluated on the testing documents. We evaluated the system by applying our simple rule-based system to the 300 testing documents from the i2b2 data set. As mentioned earlier, precision was evaluated using the micro-average, and recall using an "all-or-nothing" approach.

The recall and precision for each element of personal information were considered separately. The results in Table 8-6 and Table 8-7 apply to direct and indirect identifiers, respectively.

Table 8-6. Results of rule-based system on direct identifiers

PHI element	Precision (micro-average)	Recall (all-or-nothing)	F_2-measure (micro-average)	F_2-measure (all-or-nothing)
First name	1	0.97	0.99	0.97
Middle name	1	1	1	1
Last name	0.93	0.99	0.98	0.94
Email	1	0.99	0.99	0.99
ID	0.98	0.95	0.99	0.95
Phone number	0.93	0.98	0.97	0.97

Table 8-7. Results of rule-based system on indirect identifiers

PHI element	Precision (micro-average)	Recall (all-or-nothing)	F_2-measure (micro-average)	F_2-measure (all-or-nothing)
Date	0.95	0.90	0.97	0.92
Health care facility	1	0.99	1	0.99
Age	0.8	1	0.95	0.91
Street	1	0.78	0.83	0.81
City	0.8	0.81	0.84	0.79
State	0.8	0.9	0.88	0.87
ZIP code	1	1	1	1

For each element by itself, the overall risk levels fall below our thresholds. The precision for direct and indirect identifiers is above 70% and 80%, respectively. Recall is at or above 95% for the direct identifiers, and above 50% for indirect identifiers. Therefore, this text anonymization system would adequately manage the overall risk of disclosing the text data to Researcher Ronnie and can be used to prepare the data set for him.

What if Researcher Ronnie wanted to get a data set different from i2b2? Would this system still manage the risk adequately? There are two ways to address this question:

- Evaluate the performance of the text anonymization system on the new data set.
- Extrapolate from the i2b2 data set.

To evaluate the system on a different data set, we would need to select a sample of documents, annotate them, and then run the anonymization system on that annotated data set and evaluate the precision and recall as described earlier. If these values meet the thresholds defined for Researcher Ronnie, the rest of the documents can be anonymized using the same system and disclosed to him.

This approach is consistent with what we've been doing with structured data. Here, we would evaluate the precision and recall for the specific data set that we're working with, and decide from that whether the risk is acceptable. But the result would be specific to the data set being disclosed.

Using the second approach would be the most defensible if there were some similarity between the i2b2 data set and the new data set that Researcher Ronnie has (e.g., if they're both discharge data sets). That way there would be a strong basis for extending the results from the i2b2 evaluations to the second data set. In general, it's easier to extrapolate to other data sets when the anonymization system has been evaluated on a wide variety of data sets to begin with—i.e., data from different document types and different facilities—because people write differently in different departments and facilities.

We would like to be able to extrapolate from other data sets to decide whether we can reliably anonymize a new data set using the text anonymization system, because this makes it much easier to use the same system repeatedly. But it can be challenging to get a variety of suitable data sets to work with. You'll notice, however, that under the second approach we don't evaluate the risk for free-form text in the same way as for structured data. In the second approach we build a system that has acceptable average performance and then apply it on new data sets without further evaluation. And that's fine provided we extrapolate from similar data sets, to demonstrate that the system is reliable in the context of the data sets we want to anonymize.

Final Thoughts

Free-form text can be challenging to anonymize specifically because it's free-form, as in "anything goes:" shorthand, acronyms, nicknames, spelling errors, you name it. Text anonymization systems exist in academic literature, so it's not an insurmountable problem. But evaluating the system so that it truly meets the requirements of health care, with assurances of low risk, needs to be done in an exacting way. For direct identifiers, there's no leeway—recall, or sensitivity, needs to be around 95%. For indirect identifiers, we can use a risk-based method similar to what we did with a structured data set and evaluate the risk for our attack scenarios. This allows us to come up with a minimum recall that fits the context of our data release.

There's evidence that rule-based systems tend to have better recall than model-based systems. But model-based systems tend to have better precision. A good way to design a text anonymization system is therefore to run a rule-based first pass with a model-based second pass to improve precision. We've shown you what you can expect from a rule-based system in terms of performance. A second-pass model-based system would need only to classify detected elements as false positives or true positives.

References

1. C. van Rijsbergen, *Information Retrieval*, 2nd ed. (Oxford: Butterworth-Heinemann, 1979).

2. M. Sokolova, "Evaluation Measures for Detection of Personal Health Information," *Proceedings of the Workshop on Biomedical Natural Language Processing* in conjunction with the 8th International Conference on Recent Advances in Natural Language Processing (INCOMA, 2001), 19–26.

3. O. Ferrandez, B. South, S. Shen, F.J. Friedlin, M. Samore, and S. Meystre, "Evaluating Current Automatic De-identification Methods with Veteran's Health Administration Clinical Documents," _BMC Medical Research Methodology_ 12:(2012): 109.

4. K. El Emam, D. Buckeridge, R. Tamblyn, A. Neisa, E. Jonker, and A. Verma, "The Re-identification Risk of Canadians from Longitudinal Demographics," *BMC Medical Informatics and Decision Making* 11:1 (2011): 46.

5. P. Golle, "Revisiting the Uniqueness of Simple Demographics in the US Population," *Proceedings of the 5th ACM Workshop on Privacy in Electronic Society* (New York: ACM, 2006), 77–80.

6. GATE, A General Architecture for Text Engineering (*http://gate.ac.uk*). Natural Language Processing Group, Sheffield University.

7. Informatics for Integrating Biology and the Bedside (i2b2) (*https://www.i2b2.org*)

8. HCUP Central Distributor SID. Number of Discharges by Year (*http://1.usa.gov/discharges*). Healthcare Cost and Utilization Project (HCUP), Agency for Healthcare Research and Quality.

CHAPTER 9

Geospatial Aggregation: Dissemination Areas and ZIP Codes

Location information about patients and their providers can be used to re-identify individuals. In fact, location is often one of the critical pieces of information for a successful re-identification attack. This means that when we de-identify a data set, we need to look at the risks posed by ZIP codes and postal codes and find ways to reduce these risks.

Where patients live, where they get treatments or consultations, where they get their prescription drugs, and where they get lab tests all constitute geospatial information. And most, if not all, of this information is usually found in health databases. Even if location is missing from a data set, it can sometimes be reverse engineered or found elsewhere quite easily. If the name of the health care provider is included but location (i.e., the place of service) is missing, a simple search in the yellow pages can often get an adversary this information. Or the location of service can be found through professional bodies—the address of a physician's practice is usually available through the college if you know their name or National Provider Identifier (NPI).

However, location information is often critical for a lot of analytics.[1] Patients showing up at an emergency department with gastrointestinal problems might be from the same neighborhood or school. Maybe they all ate a bad batch of Atlantic herring at the cafeteria. In a public-health context it's important to know where these patients came from. You can't identify this cluster and zero in on the possible cause of this spike in the incidence rate of gastro bugs without it. Even researchers looking at this after the fact would want to know that there's an isolated cluster in the data, to differentiate it from baseline rates of gastro for a larger geographic area.

Where the Wild Things Are

In practice, the most commonly available geographic information is the ZIP or postal code. These characterize areas where a patient lives or receives a service. The main purpose of these codes is to organize the delivery of mail, so they change often as these areas are modified to improve the delivery of mail. More stable areas are used for the census, such as the ZIP Code Tabulation Areas (ZCTAs) in the US and dissemination areas (DAs) in Canada.

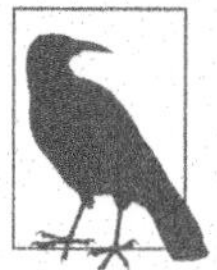

In some cases, exact locations may be available, such as a patient's address, so that longitude and latitude can then be calculated. The exact location can be selected as the center of the dwelling at that address, or the center of the street. Often the address is found, however, in free-form text. Various geocoding methods can be used to standardize, parse, and convert the address to an exact point. But often analysis is performed just on the ZIP or postal code because it's a field on its own, which makes it very easy to work with. In this chapter we'll consider only the case where areas are known, rather than exact geospatial points.

Location information is a quasi-identifier, so it needs to be de-identified when a data set is used or disclosed for secondary purposes. Like all data elements, we want to have as much detail as possible after the de-identification so that the data is meaningful for analytics. The most common way to de-identify ZIP and postal codes is through *cropping*, by retaining only the first *x* number of characters. For example, the Canadian postal code "K1L8H1" could be cropped to its three-character version "K1L," which makes sense because the "K1L" area is a superset of the "K1L8H1" area. We saw examples of such cropping when we were dealing with the BORN data set in earlier chapters. Similarly, US ZIP codes can be cropped from five digits to, say, three digits.

The biggest problem with cropping is that the cropped area may be so large that any local information is lost. The larger area characterized by the cropped location code may be useless for the type of analysis that is planned. Many cropped areas are also oddly shaped into donuts or elongated chili peppers. Of even greater concern is that an analysis of the larger, and possibly oddly shaped, area may give the wrong results by hiding important effects. Therefore, it's important that the larger (de-identified) area is the smallest possible area that will ensure that the risk of re-identification is acceptably small.

So, instead of cropping, we go about this by clustering adjacent areas into larger ones. The advantage of clustering over cropping is that we can get much smaller areas while ensuring that the risk of re-identification is below our threshold. Basically, clustering is more flexible than cropping, because we are grouping areas based on risk rather than the whims of a government service whose goal is optimizing the delivery of standard mail. The potential disadvantage is that we end up with nonstandard groupings of ZIP or postal codes—but we have ways of addressing this as well.

Being Good Neighbors

Geographic areas are represented as polygons. In order to cluster polygons, you need to be able to determine which ones are adjacent. Because the data sets health researchers deal with are quite large, you also have to be able to do this very efficiently. Otherwise it could take days, or maybe even weeks, to cluster areas for a single data set (and we've been there before).

The easiest way to determine whether two polygons are adjacent is simply to look at the points they have in common. We're not interested in two polygons that share only one point in common—what we want are polygons that share a side. So in theory, we can consider polygons that have at least two points in common. If only it were that simple!

We actually want something a bit more specific when we're looking to compare adjacent areas, because we also want to consider their size and shape. We're looking for good neighbors. Clustering a large area with a small one will simply drown out the details in the smaller area. We would rather have small areas clustered together. And we don't want to end up with really thin and long clusters, or chili peppers, because then we won't be able to pinpoint where something interesting has happened when we run our analytics.

Distance Between Neighbors

So, let's forget about those points in common between polygons and come at this problem from a different angle. A simple way to determine which polygons are close to each other is to compute the shortest distance between them. We would then cluster the polygons that are closest to one another. But this can be misleading.

Polygons A and B in Figure 9-1 are the shortest distance apart, but most of the points in these polygons are quite far apart. Polygons B and C, however, have a lot of points that are close together. If we cluster based on the shortest distance between polygons, A and B become one cluster. But it makes more sense to cluster polygons B and C together, because they have a lot of points that are close together rather than just two. One way to do that is to compute the *Hausdorff distance*.

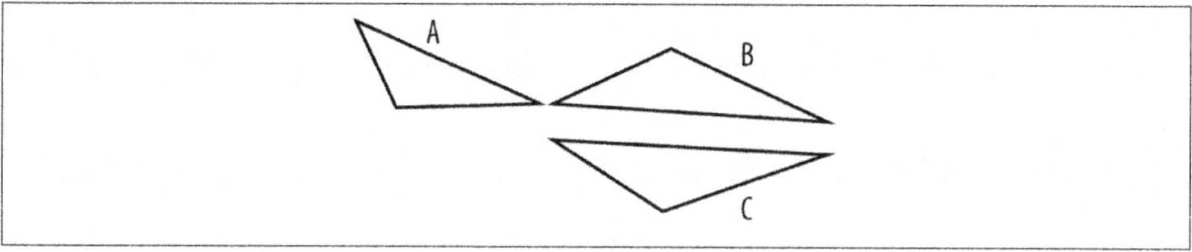

Figure 9-1. Won't you be my neighbor? Polygons A and B are closer, but B and C have more in common.

The Hausdorff distance from A to B is the distance between the furthest point in A to the closest point in B (d_1 in Figure 9-2); the Hausdorff distance from B to A is the distance between the furthest point in B to the closest point in A (d_2 Figure 9-2). Obviously the distances d_1 and d_2 (from A to B or B to A) can be different, so the Hausdorff distance of A and B is the maximum of these two distances (i.e., $\max(d_1, d_2)$).

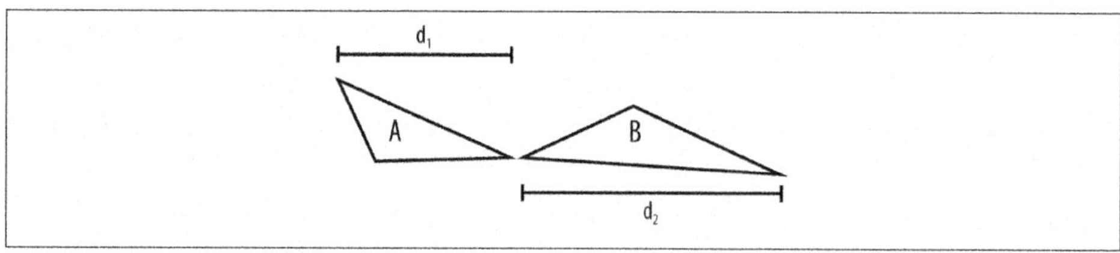

Figure 9-2. The best neighbors are close. This is how we compute the Hausdorff distance in one dimension.

Circle of Neighbors

We need to compute the Hausdorff distances among the vertices in the polygon—but geographic areas tend to be quite irregular and can have many vertices. Determining the Hausdorff distance can therefore be computationally intensive. We need to find a way to improve the approximation, and the way we'll do that is by generalizing the polygon to a circle of the same area.

The first step is to figure out the "center" of the polygon. The most obvious way to do that is to compute the centroid of the polygon, but that might not be a good representation of the center, in practical terms, because it could be at the top of a mountain or in the middle of a lake. It's better to use a "representative point," which adjusts the centroid to be closer to where the majority of the population lives and moves it away from uninhabited areas. In Canada this is quite important because most of the population lives within a short distance from the US border, and therefore a large part of the land mass is not really inhabited. Taking the centroid may result in a point that is far away from where the bulk of the population lives. National statistical agencies often produce tables with the longitude and latitude of the representative points for census areas. If the representative point is not available, we can revert to the centroid.

We can then represent each polygon by a circle of the same area as the original polygon and center it at the representative point. It's fairly straightforward to compute the area of a polygon, and for census geographies these areas are publicly available. Computing the Hausdorff distance among circles is then relatively simple. The two Ontario DAs in Figure 9-3 seem pretty close, but in Figure 9-4 they're further apart. Since the Hausdorff distance is the maximum of these two distances, it's the latter that gives us their distance. In this case, the larger area makes them farther apart, so using the Hausdorff distance meets our goal of favoring the clustering of adjacent areas that have similar sizes.

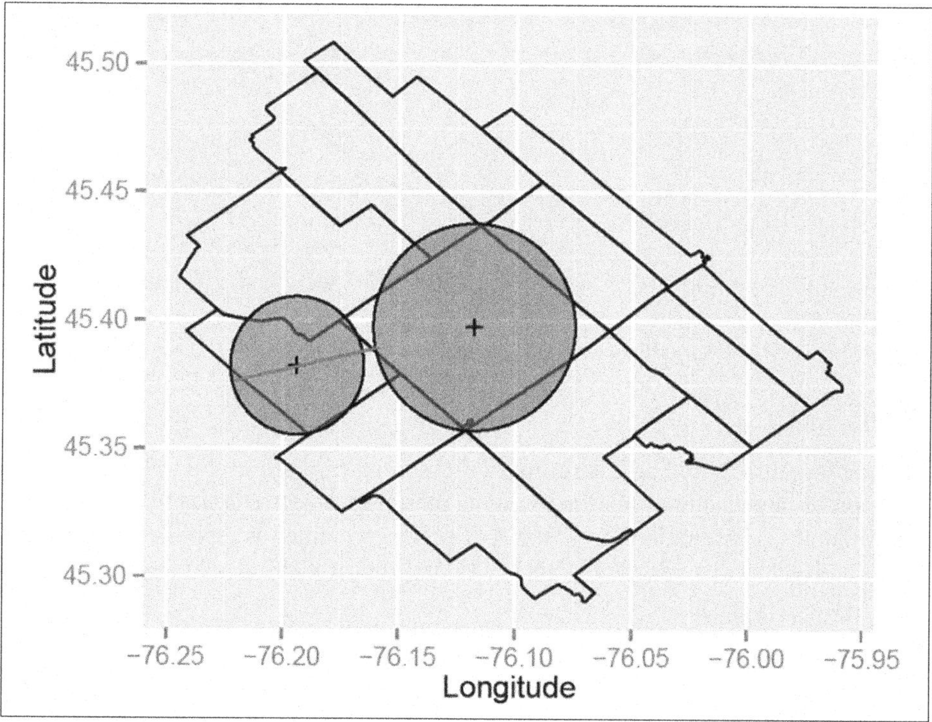

Figure 9-3. From this direction these neighbors seem close.

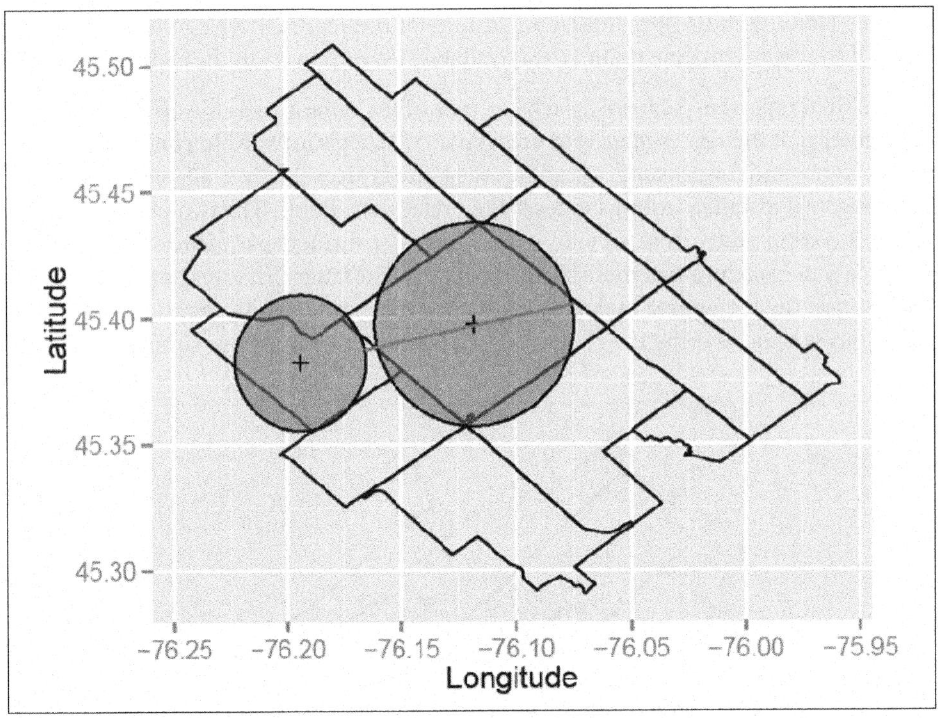

Figure 9-4. But from this direction these neighbors seem a little further apart.

Round Earth

We can't forget that the Earth is round (we're hoping this isn't up for debate), and we can improve on our approximation by taking this into account, in a way that won't affect performance. A circle on the Earth's surface can be represented as a spherical cap—think of it as a swimmer's cap on someone's head. The circle can be calculated as follows:

Radius of spherical cap

$$r = r_{earth} \times \arccos(1 - Z / 2\pi \times {r_{earth}}^2)$$

where Z is the area. While in principle the radius of the Earth depends on latitude, we'll assume that it's a constant (r_{earth}). The radius values can be precomputed for all real units beforehand and saved in a database, so the calculation doesn't affect the computation time when we do the clustering. We precomputed the radius values for all DAs in Canada, and ZCTAs in the US.

If we let our two circles be denoted by A and B, their radiuses by r_A and r_B (calculated for spherical caps), and the distance between the center of their circles by c, we get a new Hausdorff distance, this time for spherical caps:

Hausdorff for spherical caps

$$\max(c + r_A - r_B, c + r_B - r_A)$$

We haven't explained yet how to compute *c*, which is the distance between the two centroids of the circles A and B. Because the Earth is not flat (according to scientific consensus), as a starting point, we don't calculate the Euclidean distance between areas. Instead we can take into account the spherical nature of the Earth's surface, which matters more as areas get farther from the Equator.

To calculate the distance between points along the Earth's surface, we use something called the *Haversine distance*. We'll spare you the details of this equation as it is well known, except to say that it takes the latitude and longitude of two points and calculates the distance between them.

Flat Earth

It just so happens that in practice it's often much easier to work with the Euclidean distance than the Haversine distance. Being able to use the Euclidean distance allows us to implement some relatively straightforward efficiencies for large data sets. Our problem is a clustering one, which means that we only need to find the nearest neighbor to a point. We don't actually care whether the exact distances we compute are correct, so long as their ranking is correct.

The question is whether we retain the same ranks with the Euclidean distance as with the Haversine distance. So we ran a simulation to compare results between the Euclidean distance and the Haversine distance, to see whether the rankings are similar. We selected 5,000 DAs at random, calculated both distances between each DA and all of the other DAs, and then computed the Spearman correlation between the two and averaged it across the 5,000 DAs. The Spearman correlation tells us how different the rankings are using the two approaches. In total, there are 56,204 DAs in Canada. The correlation was 0.99—almost perfect—so their rankings are quite close.

This correlation may be a bit misleading, though, because when we're looking at nearest neighbors we're often interested only in the *k* nearest neighbors, where *k* is often a small number (certainly smaller than 56,204).

Our shortcut is to find the $1.5 \times k$ nearest neighbors using the Euclidean distance and then compute the Haversine distance among those. That way we need to do the more time-consuming Haversine computation only among a small subset of neighbors rather than on the whole data set. Figure 9-5 shows the accuracy of this approach. The graph was generated by evaluating the *k* nearest neighbors calculation for 5,000 randomly selected DAs for different values of *k*. For example, if we're looking for the two nearest neighbors, using our Euclidean approach will find the correct two nearest neighbors 94.5% of the time. At the threshold of about five nearest neighbors, the Euclidean approach settles at 98% accuracy. (Note that this approximation may not work as well in other jurisdictions.)

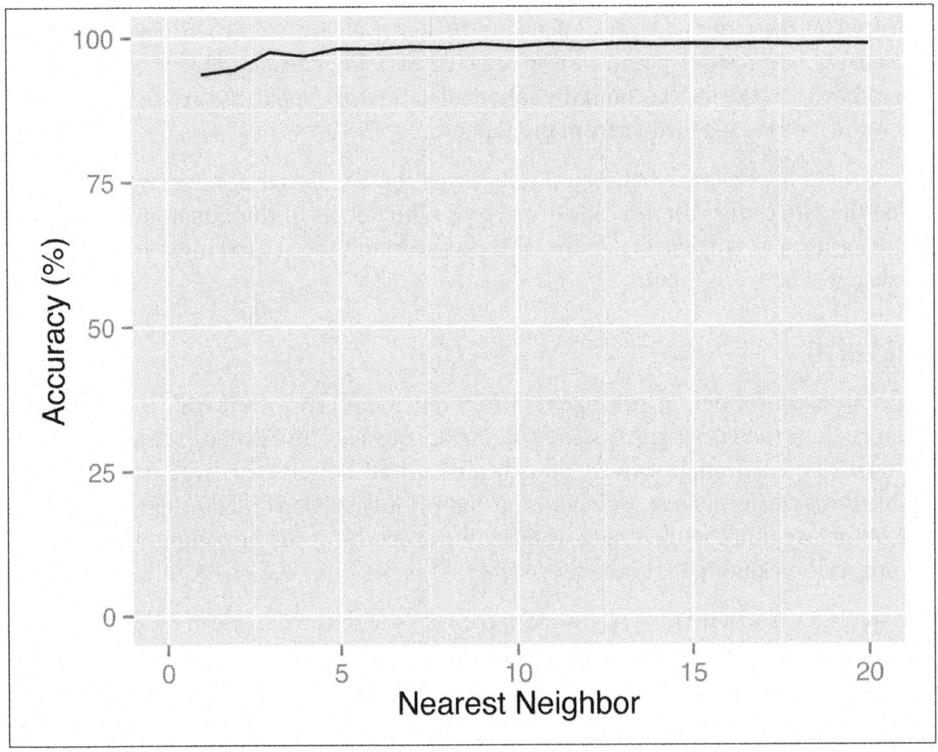

Figure 9-5. In this case the Flat Earth Society gets it close enough—the accuracy of using the Euclidean distance instead of the Haversine distance for Canadian DAs is quite high.

Clustering Neighbors

Now that we've figured out who our neighbors are, and we can do so quickly, we need to figure out which to cluster into larger areas. There are many clustering algorithms, from simple hierarchical ones to more complex graph-based ones. We won't discuss clustering in general because there are so many standard tools for doing this; rather, we'll focus on some of the techniques needed to do this clustering efficiently for geospatial data.

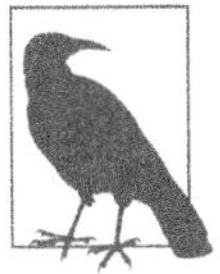

All clustering approaches that are applicable here need to have some objective function to optimize. This consists of two criteria: first, finding the smallest cluster; and second, making sure the overall risk metric, whether maximum or average, is below the threshold (earlier in the book, in Chapter 2, we discuss how to set the re-identification risk threshold). So, if we have two ways to cluster our data that are both below the re-identification risk threshold, we choose the one that has the smallest cluster sizes.

A good place to start for clustering algorithms is *k*-means. The *k*-means algorithm "grows" clusters from the individual observations, and iterates through two steps, assignment and update, until it reaches a stopping point. During the assignment step a decision is made about which cluster to group an area into. Then various metrics are calculated. The re-identification risk can be computed as part of the metrics, and that can be used to make a decision during the assignment step about whether to stop growing clusters or not.

Consider the clustering example in Figure 9-6. Here we have a DA (the grey area in the middle) that was clustered with a group of other DAs that were adjacent to it. When this data is released, we would replace the original DA with one of the DAs in that cluster. There were 11 DAs in the cluster, so each one of them (including the original DA) has a 1/11 probability of being selected as the replacement DA. This process effectively shifts the original DA to another close DA within a defined cluster that was created to meet the re-identification risk threshold. The better the clustering algorithm, the smaller this cluster will be and the smaller this shifting will be.

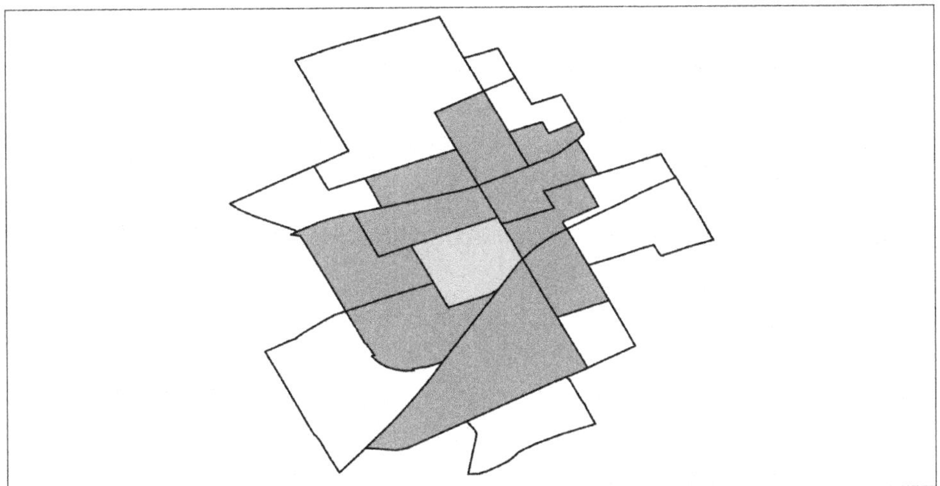

Figure 9-6. A DA is clustered with its neighbors.

We All Have Boundaries

In practice, we need to take pre-existing boundaries into account when we cluster areas. Say the data will be used by a regional public health unit. That unit has authority over a particular area with a well-defined boundary. If some outbreak is detected in an adjacent area that it doesn't have authority over, it won't be able to intervene. It's a waste of this public health unit's time to cluster areas across its boundaries. We're always striving to ensure de-identified data is of the highest utility to users, and this is just another example of that.

We can also cluster within a cropping region. If we find through de-identification that the appropriate cropping for ZIP codes is to three digits, the three-digit ZIP codes would define the boundaries we use. The clustering could then reduce the size of the areas within the three-digit ZIP code boundaries. This way we guarantee that clustering will produce an area that is at most the same size as that produced by cropping, but likely smaller, with the same re-identification risk.

Fast Nearest Neighbor

Finding the nearest neighbor is easy in a small data set. We just compute the distance between each area and all of the other areas, and sort the distances—so we need to construct an adjacency matrix. This won't work for large data sets, though. The number of distances that need to be computed is $n(n-1)/2$, where n is the number of unique areas in the data set. This scales quadratically as the data set size increases. For a data set with 10,000 unique areas, this would amount to almost 50 million computations. We need to find a more efficient way to do this!

One simple approach to finding the nearest neighbor is to use a *Hilbert curve*,[2] like the one in Figure 9-7. This is a fractal space-filling curve that allows us to project two-dimensional x,y values onto a single dimension (the Hilbert curve itself). There are other space-filling curves, but we'll only consider this one for simplicity. Points that are close in the multidimensional space should be close on the Hilbert curve as well. Then we just search above and below any point along the Hilbert curve to get its nearest neighbors. This can be very fast as it involves far fewer comparisons than creating a full adjacency matrix. But it isn't perfect—some points that are physically close to each other will be far apart on the Hilbert curve.

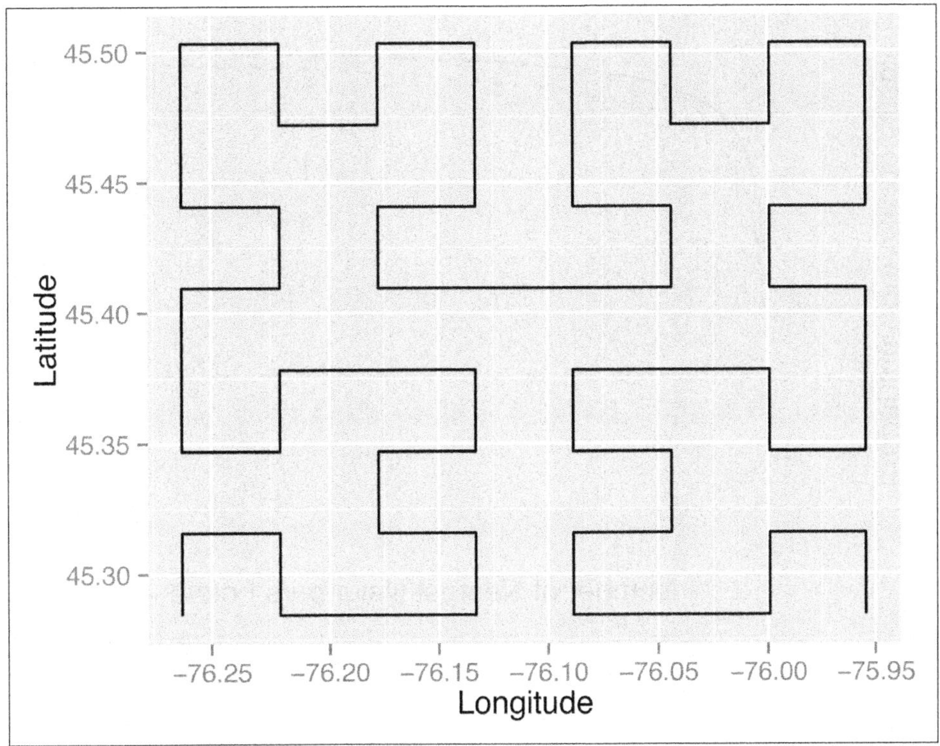

Figure 9-7. Fill it up! This is an example of a third-order Hilbert curve. The higher the order, the more space it fills in.

We evaluated the utility of the Hilbert curve to efficiently find nearest neighbors for geographic areas. We took all DAs in Canada and ZIP codes in the US, and for each compared the nearest neighbors on the Hilbert curve to the true nearest neighbors (taking into account the curvature of the Earth). The results are in Figure 9-8. Within the number of nearest neighbors along the Hilbert curve, we computed the exact distance to find the true nearest neighbors. So if we consider the 50 nearest neighbors along the Hilbert curve to a point, then the exact distance is computed between the point and those other 50 neighbors found using the Hilbert curve. This is much faster than the naive approach because now we only need to compute $n \times 50$ distances instead of $n(n-1)/2$ distances (although there are fewer when boundaries are considered).

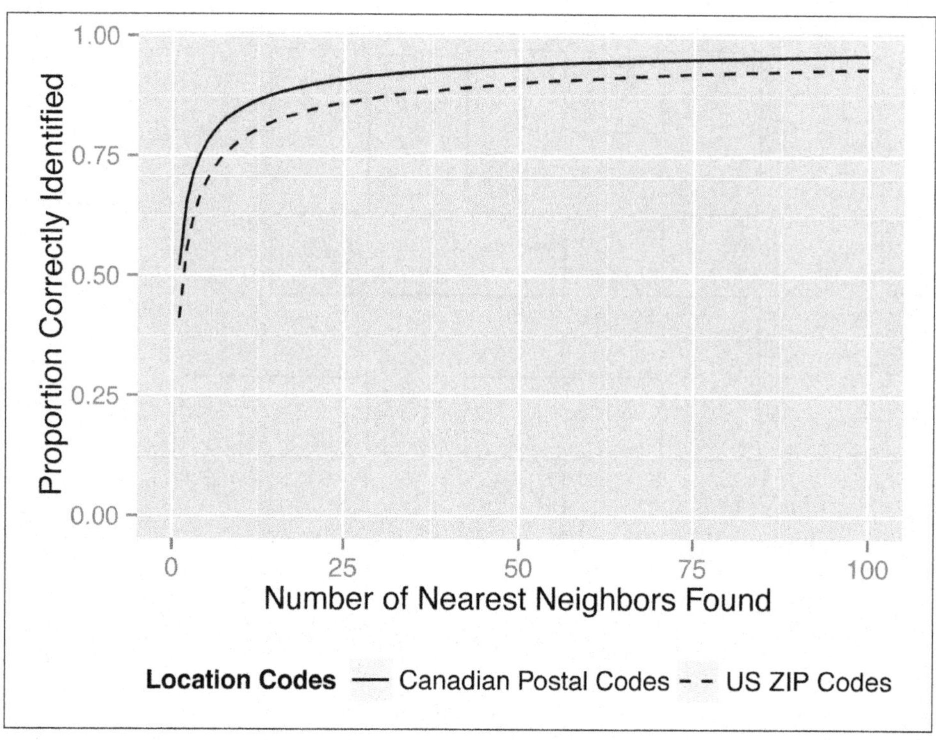

Figure 9-8. Finding the nearest neighbor with a third-order Hilbert curve. The probability of finding the true nearest neighbor increases the more Hilbert-nearest neighbors we consider.

In terms of performance, the Hilbert curve approach to clustering is great. The points on the curve can be computed once and stored in a database, so initial distance calculations would just require a very fast lookup. If more accurate results are needed, an *r*-tree could be used to compute the distances during the clustering process. This has some cost in terms of initially setting up the tree, but the lookups can be quite efficient afterwards.

Too Close to Home

Health data sets often contain multiple variables indicating location. Just as with other kinds of health information, location information tends to be correlated. Patients typically go to a doctor's office and local community pharmacy that is near their home. This means that even if we suppress, crop, or cluster data on the patient location, an adversary might be able to recover that information from knowledge of where the provider or pharmacy is located.

There's a lot of evidence on the distance between patient residence and where they receive medical services. Location, or spatial accessibility,[3] is an important factor in accessing health care as increased travel time for patients often presents as a barrier to access. Medical geographers are working to address accessibility issues with models to manage the amount of travel required to access services.

Not surprisingly, the evidence suggests that the majority of patients live within a reasonable distance to their health care provider. However, what "reasonable" means in this context is subject to debate. In North America, travel distances and times vary considerably but the threshold for greater vs. lesser travel burden seems to hover between a distance of 30 and 80 kilometers (20 and 50 miles) and a time of 30 minutes.[4, 5, 6, 7] This evidence also suggests that patients receiving specialized care tend to travel longer distances, as opposed to those going to general practice and visiting family doctors. Patients aslo tend to live closer to their pharmacies,[8, 9, 10, 11] and individuals living in rural areas tend to travel longer distances to get care.[12, 13, 14]

When provider or pharmacy information can reveal information about a patient's location, we call this a *geoproxy* attack. Many data sets include provider information, in the form of the provider or prescriber's name, NPI number, or DEA number. Community pharmacy names or ZIP codes can also be used for geoproxy attacks.

There are, of course, exceptions. Sometimes the drugs are dispensed from mailing centers to the providers or to special clinics that perform, say, injections. In those cases the pharmacy information cannot be used for geoproxy attacks because it's not indicative of patient location.

Levels of Geoproxy Attacks

There are different levels of geoproxy attacks. For example, we can have a geoproxy attack on a record by using the provider or pharmacy ZIP code in that record to predict the patient's ZIP code. Or, if we have a claims data set where each record is a claim, we can have a geoproxy attack on the set of claims. This is a *record* geoproxy attack.

On another level of attack, the adversary uses the information from multiple records. If a patient has 50 claims and these claims cover visits to three different providers, an adversary can use the ZIP code from these three providers to predict where the patient lives. This attack would use some form of triangulation strategy to compute the most likely patient ZIP code given the visits to providers in these three other locations. This is a *patient* geoproxy attack. It's probably more informative than a record-level attack because, at the end of the day, an adversary would want to know the patient's ZIP code.

Of course, the risks will vary by data set. In some data sets, the ability to predict patient ZIP code is quite high, whereas in others it's much lower (although it's never zero). It's something that needs to be evaluated for each data set.

There are at least four variants of a patient geoproxy attack, each using a different approach to account for provider location in the triangulation process (we'll use a claims data set to illustrate the differences):

- Each *claim* is kept as a record. This means that if ten claims are made during the same visit to the same provider, they will show up as ten records in the data set with the same ZIP code. This causes ZIP codes where the patient has had multiple claims to be weighted more heavily than ZIP codes where only a single claim is made.
- Each *provider visit* results in a record for the corresponding patient, no matter how many claims the patient makes in a single visit. This causes ZIP codes where the patient has seen a single provider multiple times to be weighted more heavily than ZIP codes where a provider is seen only once.
- Each *provider* results in a single record for the corresponding patient, no matter how many times the patient has visited that provider. This causes ZIP codes where the patient has seen many providers to be weighted more heavily than ZIP codes where only a single provider is seen.
- Each *provider ZIP code* results in a single record for the corresponding patient, no matter how many distinct providers in that ZIP code that patient has visited. ZIP codes where the patient has seen many providers are therefore weighted equally to ZIP codes where only a single provider is seen.

To illustrate how to measure geoproxy risk, we'll look at the third variant, with distinct providers. On balance this makes the most sense since it's more likely that a patient lives close to where they have the most providers, given the evidence we described in "Too Close to Home" on page 142.

Measuring Geoproxy Risk

Let's measure the geoproxy risk in an insurance claims data set from the state of Louisiana. We have already looked at this data set in other chapters. The data contains patient and provider ZIP codes. We want to determine the probability of using the provider's location to accurately predict the patient's location. Because we have patient ZIP codes, we can compute the actual probability.

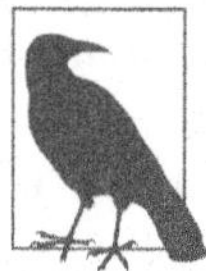

Geoproxy risk can be taken into account during the measurement of re-identification risk. If it's too high, you might find it necessary to apply transformations to the provider information as well as the patient data.

When measuring geoproxy risk, we need to make an assumption about the adversary —the number of nearest neighbors that the adversary will use. For simplicity, let's just consider a record geoproxy attack. For example, an adversary can say that the patient's five-digit ZIP code is exactly the same as the provider's five-digit ZIP code. In this case, the adversary doesn't use any neighbors at all to make that prediction (i.e., the adversary uses zero nearest neighbors).

Let's say that a provider has a practice at ZIP code *G*. All other ZIP codes can be ranked in terms of how close they are to *G*. The ZIP code with rank 1 is the closest to *G*, the one with rank 2 is the second closest, and so on. We saw earlier in this chapter how to measure the distance between two ZIP codes.

An adversary can then assume that the patient is in the same ZIP code as the provider, or in the next nearest neighbor (i.e., the ZIP code with rank 1). In this case, the adversary will have two ZIP codes that the patient can live in, and has to guess which one it is. So the probability of predicting correctly is at most 0.5. Similarly, the adversary can consider the two nearest neighbors, in which case he has to guess which one of three ZIP codes the patient lives in. Therefore, the accuracy of an adversary's geoproxy attack will depend on how many nearest neighbors are considered. More nearest neighbors means more confusion, and a lower chance of guessing the right one (unless there's an effective way to weigh those nearest neighbors to pinpoint the right one).

To triangulate the patient ZIP code from multiple provider ZIP codes, we start by finding the 50 nearest ZIP codes for each provider's ZIP code. Points are then given to each neighbor, equal to 50 minus the rank of its ZIP code with respect to the identified provider's ZIP code. Therefore, the provider's ZIP code (0) receives 50 points, the nearest neighbor (1) 49 points, and so on down to 1 point for the 49th-nearest neighbor. This process is repeated for each provider associated with the patient. The sum of the points allocated to each ZIP code is the score for that ZIP code.

To evaluate the effectiveness of our triangulation approach, we need a way to compare the patient's real ZIP code to the triangulated ZIP codes. We do this by ranking the patient's real ZIP code based on its score compared to those of the triangulated ZIP codes (i.e., seeing how many ZIP codes have a higher score than the patient's real one). So, if the patient's true ZIP code has a score of 240, and there are four other ZIP codes that have been given a higher score, the patient's ZIP code has a rank of 4.

In reality, we would often be releasing the data set with ZIP codes that are correct to within a certain number of digits. Recall that a common way to release ZIP code information is to crop it. But even if geospatial clustering is used, the clusters are created within some predefined political or service delivery boundaries. When scoring the ZIP codes closest to a provider, an adversary can just assign zero points to those that are not in the same cropped ZIP code.

To illustrate this point, let's look at the table with two records in Table 9-1. Here the data set is being released with the three-digit ZIP code of the patient and the five-digit ZIP code of the provider. Predicted patient ZIP codes that fall outside of their true three-digit ZIP code are discarded because we know they're wrong. Therefore, in our example, we limit our predictions of the patient's ZIP code to those starting with 956.

Table 9-1. An example of patient and provider ZIP code being released

Patient ZIP3	Provider ZIP5
956	95688
956	95601

We computed the average geoproxy risk for predicting patient location from provider location, using the triangulation approach just described, for the claims data from the state of Louisiana. The results are shown in Figure 9-9. We considered different situations where the patient's ZIP code was also being released, from four-digit ZIP codes down to no patient ZIP codes being released at all (zero-digit ZIP codes). We implemented this by just dropping the ZIP codes that were not within the boundary from the score calculation. As expected, the adversary's best guess is the highest-ranked location, and more patient ZIP code digits being released leads to a higher probability of predicting the patient's real ZIP code.

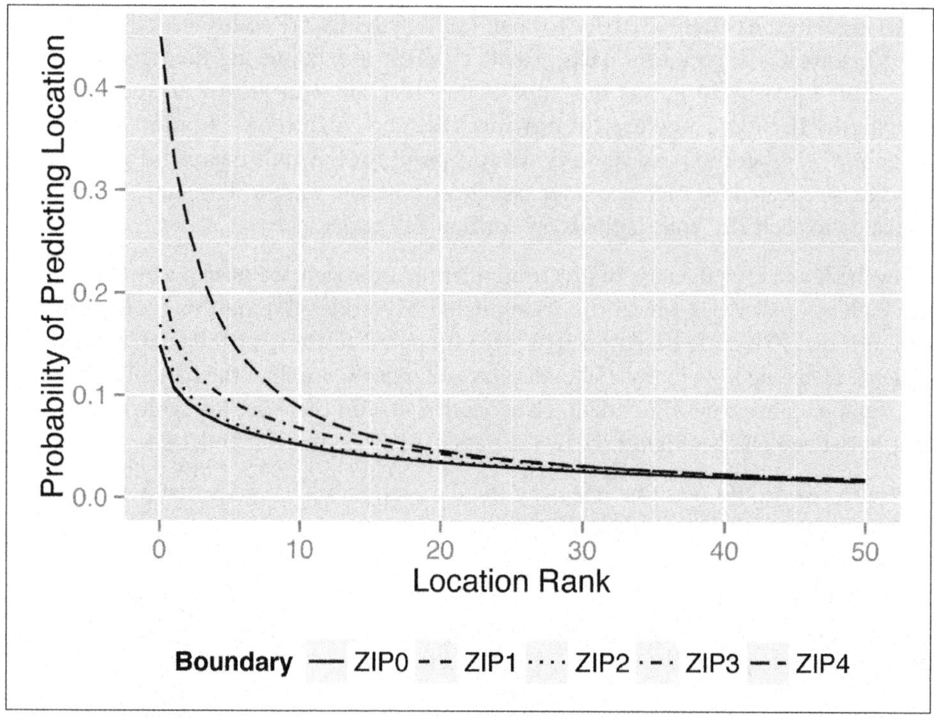

Figure 9-9. The average geoproxy risk for the claims data set from the state of Louisiana.

But there are more sophisticated methods that can be used to predict patient location, although they're typically more computationally intensive. We've implemented the Gi* algorithm, that is normally used for hot-spot detection. The algorithm returns, for each region considered, a z-score that reflects the likelihood that the local cluster of points is due to chance.

The Gi* algorithm requires a value (x_i) for each region, and a spatial weight ($w_{i,j}$) reflecting the distance between regions i and j. For the regional value, we use the total number of patient-provider interactions at that region. For the spatial weight, we use the inverse Hausdorff distance with a zone of indifference of 10km. Therefore, any distance less than 10km will receive a spatial weight of 0.1, and larger distances will get a smaller weight.

The results using the Gi* algorithm increase the probability of predicting location by about 0.05 over those presented in Figure 9-9. But all these results assume that the adversary is trying to predict the patient's five-digit ZIP code. That's not always going to be the case. The adversary could try to predict, say, the three-digit ZIP code of the patient instead. But the same approaches described can be used to predict the geoproxy risk of these attacks as well.

Accounting for Geoproxy Risk

Now that we're able to compute geoproxy risk, how can we incorporate it into the overall risk measurement? Let's consider the situation where we release the patient's three-digit ZIP code, and the five-digit ZIP codes of their providers. We don't know that a geoproxy attack will always result in a higher risk of re-identification. Therefore, we need to consider the risk or re-identification with and without geoproxy risk, and ensure we manage the one with the highest risk.

Without a geoproxy attack, we only need the patient's three-digit ZIP code (along with all their other quasi-identifiers), and we ignore the ZIP codes of their providers. In this case the risk is measured the same as we've done before. For attack T1, for example, we would compute:

Attack T1

$Pr(\text{re-id, attempt}) = Pr(\text{attempt}) \times Pr(\text{re-id} \mid \text{attempt})$

where $Pr(\text{re-id} \mid \text{attempt})$ uses the three-digit ZIP code as a quasi-identifier.

When we include a geoproxy attack, we use the patient's five-digit ZIP code (along with all their other quasi-identifiers), and we use the ZIP codes of their providers to predict the patient's five-digit ZIP code. We then compute following conditional probability:

Attack T1 (Geoproxy)

$Pr(\text{re-id, attempt, geoproxy}) = Pr(\text{attempt}) \times Pr(\text{geoproxy} \mid \text{attempt}) \times Pr(\text{re-id} \mid \text{attempt, geoproxy})$

The term *Pr*(geoproxy | attempt) acknowledges that the five-digit ZIP code is not going to be predicted correctly all the time. As an example, take the following values computed from the Louisiana data set:

- Attack T1: *Pr*(re-id, attempt) = 0.4 × 0.25 = 0.1.
- Attack T1 (Geoproxy): *Pr*(re-id | attempt, geoproxy) = 0.4 × 0.26 × 0.8 = 0.08.

As you can see from these values, the risk of re-identification using a geoproxy attack is less than the risk of re-identification *not* using a geoproxy attack. This illustrates that a geoproxy attack is not always beneficial for the adversary. In practice, though, both versions need to be considered and the highest risk is the one that's used.

Final Thoughts

Geospatial information is critical for data analytics. However, geospatial information can also increase the risk of re-identification significantly. Traditionally, basic cropping is used to generalize geographic areas, such as cropping the five-digit ZIP code to a three-digit one. This is a rather crude approach that results in losing a lot of geographic detail.

A better way is to cluster adjacent areas. This produces areas that are much smaller, and data sets that are quite realistic in comparison to the original data sets.

One last thing to consider when dealing with geospatial information is geoproxy attacks. These are instances where patient location information can be inferred from provider or pharmacy information. If the geoproxy risk has a significant impact on the overall risk of re-identification, additional transformations may need to be performed on the provider (or pharmacy) information.

References

1. K. El Emam and E. Moher, "Biomedical Data Privacy: Problems, Perspectives, and Recent Advances," *Journal of Law, Medicine & Ethics* 41:1 (2013): 37-41

2. H. Sagan, *Space-Filling Curves* (New York: Springer-Verlag, 1994).

3. M. F. Guagliardo, "Spatial accessibility of primary care: concepts, methods and challenges," Int. J. Health Geogr., vol. 3, no. 1, p. 3, 2004.

4. L. Chan, L. G. Hart, and D. C. Goodman, "Geographic Access to Health Care for Rural Medicare Beneficiaries," J. Rural Health, vol. 22, no. 2, pp. 140–146, 2006.

5. R. K. Jones and J. Jerman, "How Far Did US Women Travel for Abortion Services in 2008?," J. Womens Health, vol. 22, no. 8, pp. 706–713, Aug. 2013.

6. J. Fortney, K. Rost, M. Zhang, and J. Warren, "The Impact of Geographic Accessibility on the Intensity and Quality of Depression Treatment," Med. Care, vol. 37, no. 9, pp. 884–893, 1999.

7. D. E. Fixler, W. N. Nembhard, P. Xu, M. K. Ethen, and M. A. Canfield, "Effect of Acculturation and Distance From Cardiac Center on Congenital Heart Disease Mortality," Pediatrics, vol. 129, no. 6, pp. 1118–1124, May 2012.

8. L. Chan, L. G. Hart, and D. C. Goodman, "Geographic Access to Health Care for Rural Medicare Beneficiaries," J. Rural Health, vol. 22, no. 2, pp. 140–146, 2006.

9. D. M. Triller, J. Donnelly, and J. Rugge, "Travel-Related Savings Through a Rural, Clinic-Based Automated Drug Dispensing System," J. Community Health, vol. 30, no. 6, pp. 467–476, Dec. 2005.

10. R. Hiscock, J. Pearce, T. Blakely, and K. Witten, "Is Neighborhood Access to Health Care Provision Associated with Individual-Level Utilization and Satisfaction?," Health Serv. Res., vol. 43, no. 6, pp. 2183–2200, Dec. 2008.

11. S.-J. Lin, "Access to Community Pharmacies by the Elderly in Illinois: A Geographic Information Systems Analysis," J. Med. Syst., vol. 28, no. 3, pp. 301–309, 2004.

12. J. C. Probst, S. B. Laditka, J.-Y. Wang, and A. O. Johnson, "Effects of Residence and Race on Burden of Travel for Care: Cross Sectional Analysis of the 2001 US National Household Travel Survey," BMC Health Serv. Res., vol. 7, no. 1, p. 40, 2007.

13. K. B. Stitzenberg, E. R. Sigurdson, B. L. Egleston, R. B. Starkey, and N. J. Meropol, "Centralization of Cancer Surgery: Implications for Patient Access to Optimal Care," J. Clin. Oncol., vol. 27, no. 28, pp. 4671–4678, Aug. 2009.

14. F. Brundisini, M. Giacomini, D. DeJean, M. Vanstone, K. Winsor, and A. Smith, "Chronic Disease Patients' Experiences with Accessing Health Care in Rural and Remote Areas: A Systematic Review and Qualitative Meta-Synthesis," Ont. Health Technol. Assess. Ser., vol. 13, no. 15, pp. 1–33, 2013.

CHAPTER 10

Medical Codes: A Hackathon

There are a few standard coding systems used in health data, for procedures, diseases, and drugs. We've mentioned them a few times already, but a chapter about codes sounds pretty boring. Well, we're not about to list the codes and leave it at that. You can get books about these codes elsewhere (and they are oh, so interesting to read… to be fair, they're references, not books to curl up with in an armchair). No, what we'll look at are the specific ways to anonymize these codes in health data. By now you know the drill: generalization and suppression. But—spoiler alert—we have another trick up our sleeve to keep the original codes within generalized groups. This is a major aid in increasing the utility of data. But we'll save that one for last, just to add to the anticipation.

We had the chance to apply all of these methods to a data set used for a hackathon known as the Cajun Code Fest[1] (how awesome is that name?). A hackathon is a competition in which programmers are (figuratively) caged up in some common space to code day and night to accomplish a predefined goal (no programmers were harmed in the making of this hackathon). For the Cajun Code Fest, in Lafayette, Louisiana, registrants were given de-identified claims data for the state and told to come up with something that would improve health care.

Taking advantage of health data requires more than just programming skills, so the organizers of the Cajun Code Fest encouraged people who had knowledge of health care to take part, even if they knew nothing about programming. Once people arrived, they would be put into multidisciplinary teams. This hackathon is probably the best example of health data being made available for all the right reasons. Competitors also got to enjoy the Festival International de Louisiane, with music and—it should go without saying in the South—lots of food (will code for crawfish!). A hackathon is a fun and engaging way to get people involved, as the Cajun Code Fest proves.

Codes in Practice

The point of medical codes is not to provide clarity to human readers, at least not directly, because they look a lot like random alphanumeric strings. What they do is standardize medical categories assigned and consumed by health data users. And they are very precise. Usually, health data sets will place the code and its individual description in adjacent fields (the description itself is human readable, although it will sometimes be in short form or be terse in order to keep the text field to a minimum number of characters).

Let's look at the most common sets of coding systems we see in medical data. If you have something different in your data, don't fret. The methods we'll look at can be applied to different coding systems, or be mapped to these coding systems:

International Classification of Diseases (ICD)
: This system, maintained by the World Health Organization (WHO), provides diagnostic codes for classifying diseases, as well as signs, symptoms, complaints, and external causes of diseases or injuries. It's extremely detailed, with literally thousands of codes arranged in a hierarchy that we can take advantage of for anonymization. The US uses ICD-9 with a Clinical Modification (ICD-9-CM), which includes procedures.[2] But the ICD-9 system (which has about 14,000 disease codes and 4,000 procedure codes) is about 30 years old, and most countries have already adopted ICD-10 (which has about 10 times more codes!). US providers will be required to use ICD-10-CM about a year after this book goes to press, if there are no delays.

Common Procedural Terminology (CPT)
: Maintained (and copyright protected) by the American Medical Association (AMA), this coding system is used to describe medical, surgical, and diagnostic services in the US.[3] It's primarily used for billing purposes, with about 8,000 codes, so we see it in claims data all the time. Similar to the ICD system, the system is hierarchical, which we'll make use of in anonymization. Healthcare Common Procedure Coding System (HCPCS) codes are often included in the same field as CPT codes. Once ICD-10 codes are adopted in the US, CPT and HCPCS codes will continue to be used in outpatient and office settings (whereas ICD-10-CM will be used for inpatient procedures).

National Drug Code (NDC)
: This is the coding system used in the US to identify drug products. You can think of the NDC as a serial number for a drug product, given by the Food and Drug Administration (FDA), which will change for different manufacturers and distributors, different doses, and different forms of the drug (e.g., liquid, pill, or inhaler). In order to manage the risk of identity disclosure from drug information, anyone anonymizing data also needs to generalize NDCs into a hierarchy, which they don't

have. WHO has a system we can map these to for the sake of anonymization? No, wait, we mean the WHO has such a system, thankfully.

The Cajun Code Fest included all the coding systems just described in the competition data. The introductory webcast to discuss the competition and, specifically, the data that competitors would have access to gave the frequency of the top diseases, procedures, and drugs. The slides were then posted online for anyone to read. This might not sound like a big deal, but it means that those particular codes could not be given in a generalized form, or suffer a lot of suppression, and that masking could not change the frequency of those codes.

Here's why. Imagine that we mapped code 410 to 414 to mask the original code. Well, that won't work because an adversary could use the frequency of code 410 provided in the documentation to figure out that code 414 is in fact 410 (i.e., a frequency attack). So we needed something a little smarter to de-identify the data and preserve its utility.

Generalization

Normally generalization wouldn't work here because, as we just explained, we needed to preserve the original codes. If we grouped ICD-9-CM codes from 410 to 414 into Myocardial Infarction, the original codes would be lost. But we're not about to throw out the baby with the bathwater. We need generalization to group like codes together. An adversary is unlikely to know the exact codes that a patient has in her data (because they're so very detailed and precise).

Remember that we said there are literally thousands of ICD-9 codes—the same applies to the other codes as well. So whether we're going to produce generalized groups in place of the original codes or not, we still need generalization. This is something we need to apply somewhat differently to each coding system (although the common thread is having a hierarchy to work with).

The Digits of Diseases

Let's focus primarily on ICD-9-CM codes, since that's what we had for the Cajun Code Fest, and they're still used in the US. ICD-9 disease codes are five digits long and are arranged in a hierarchy. More digits means more precision. The fewest number of digits you'll see for disease codes in their original form is three (codes below 100 will be padded with zeros to keep the length to three). Then there's supposed to be a period (although some data sets drop the period), and one or two more optional digits meant to define the disease in more precision.

Our first level of generalization for ICD-9 codes is therefore the three-digit codes, made up of the first three digits of the original code (this is something we've evaluated elsewhere).[4] A higher level of generalization would be two-digit codes (using the first two digits of the original code), and then even higher would be one-digit codes (the first digit of the original code, of course). It's not perfect, and some will argue with the diagnostic accuracy of this generalization approach, but it's quick to implement. Three digits also works for E and V codes (external causes of injury and supplemental classification), and procedure codes can use the first two digits instead (all part of the clinical modification). This can get a bit confusing, so let's focus on disease codes.

For an even better generalization than three-digit ICD-9 codes, one that offers more or less the same number of disease and procedure categories but better diagnostic precision, there's the publicly available dictionary produced by a team at Vanderbilt.[5] The Vanderbilt ICD-9 code groups were developed for Phenome-Wide Association Studies (PheWAS), and loosely follow the three-digit category and section groupings defined with the ICD-9 code system itself. For the Cajun Code Fest, we started with these code groups (see Table 10-1).

Table 10-1. Three's company when it comes to ICD-9 disease codes. Broader generalizations that group ranges of ICD–9 codes are provided by the definitions in the ICD-9 codebook.[2]

Level of generalization	Description	Example
ICD-9 chapter definition	Broad 3-digit group	Diseases of the circulatory system (390–459)
ICD-9 section definition	3-digit group	Ischemic heart disease (410–414)
3 digits	Minimum ICD-9 code	Other acute and subacute forms (411)
4/5 digits	Subclassification	Acute coronary occlusion without myocardial infarction (411.81)

Really, to generalize ICD-9 codes more broadly than with three-digit codes, it's probably better to move up the generalization hierarchy using the Clinical Classifications Software (CCS). As odd as the name may be, CCS is actually a system for grouping diseases and procedures into clinically meaningful categories, developed as part of the Healthcare Cost and Utilization Project (HCUP).[6] This is more sophisticated than simply cropping ICD-9 codes and will produce more meaningful data than ICD-9 section definitions. We won't discuss the use of CCS as a generalization scheme in this book any more than this, but it's worth knowing that it's out there in case you ever need it.

ICD sections further attempt to group like diseases into broad categories. Alternatively primary condition groups can be used to gather like diseases into broad categories, a generalization scheme we've used before (diseases are grouped into 45 broad diagnostic categories based on relative similarity and mortality rates).[7] But this raises an important point, because primary condition groups were created in part because health experts don't necessarily agree with the way some codes are grouped in the ICD-9 hierarchy. Like CCS, we won't discuss these further, but see the references if you ever you need a broader generalization scheme than what ICD-9 codes provide.[8]

So really we have three generalizations we can use to produce meaningful health data, depending on how much we need to reduce risk: Vanderbilt ICD-9 code groups, CCS, and primary condition groups. That isn't to say we can't use cropping, or ICD-9 section definitions, but these three generalizations are better in terms of preserving the utility of the data for analytics.

The Digits of Procedures

CPT codes are similar to ICD-9 codes: they're five digits long, although we can, and most often do, use three digits for generalization. There are also 17 broad CPT categories that sometimes have to be used in cases where the risk of re-identification for the data set is much higher than the risk threshold. Another option, as with ICD-9 codes, is to crop at the second, or even first, digit of the code.

Unfortunately, because CPT codes are exclusively used in claims data for the purposes of billing, and they are copyright protected (i.e., you have to pay to use them), they simply aren't seen much in research. As a result, we haven't seen any other dictionaries available to generalize them differently since researchers haven't developed grouping systems for CPT codes. So, there's not much more we can say about them here.

The (Alpha)Digits of Drugs

The NDC system used in the US doesn't have a hierarchy, so we need to map the codes to something we can work with. We already mentioned that the WHO has such a system, called the Anatomic Therapeutic Chemical (ATC) classification. This system provides a hierarchy for drug utilization research,[9] but we can take advantage of this hierarchy for our own purposes. We're sure they won't mind, given that our purposes are genuinely for the greater good. And like the ICD, the ATC is a publicly available resource.

The ATC classification system is divided into 14 main anatomical groups, depending on the organ or system on which the drug is meant to act (e.g., blood and blood-forming organs). The main groups are followed by therapeutic, pharmacological, and chemical subgroups, before coding the chemical substance.

Although drugs are "classified according to the main therapeutic use of the main active ingredient," this classification structure implies that a drug can be given multiple ATC codes depending on how it's used. And similar to ICD and CPT codes, we truncate the codes to generalize them based on their hierarchy. The equivalent to three-digit ICD-9 or CPT codes is, in this case, a four-character ATC code (see the example in Table 10-2).

Table 10-2. This is your brain on ATC codes. Similar to ICD codes, but for drugs. Let's break down C01DA02, which is used to treat heart disease.

Level	Code type	Description	Example
1	1 letter	Anatomical group	C for cardiovascular
2	2 digits	Therapeutic group	01 for cardiac therapy
3	1 letter	Therapeutic/pharmacological subgroup	D for vasodilators
4	1 letter	Chemical/therapeutic/pharmacological subgroup	A for organic nitrates

Level	Code type	Description	Example
5	2 digits	Chemical substance	02 for glyceryl trinitrate

Although the WHO is an international body, it doesn't provide a dictionary for mapping from a specific country's drug code system to its own—it's up to countries themselves to do this. Because the ATC classification system is mainly used for research, the FDA hasn't provided a map from the NDC system. And digital pharma systems used by pharmacies haven't provided this dictionary either, at least as far as we know. So, we developed our own conversion table from NDCs to ATC codes that we'll use until something better comes along.[10]

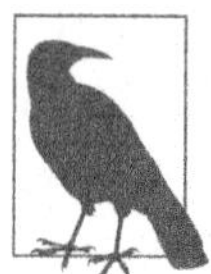

Converting NDCs to ATC codes requires knowledge of pharmaceutical drugs to differentiate between generic names, routes of administration, and main anatomical groups, as well as knowing where to find relevant information.

We had a team of six pharmacy employees that independently participated in this work, and they all commented that the combination drugs, those with multiple active ingredients, were the most difficult to map. All the same, they ended up with almost perfect agreement on a sample of codes.

With every data set we work with, however, we need to convert more NDCs over to the ATC classification system, both because there will be different drugs used in different jurisdictions, for different insurance providers, different populations, etc., and also because of the way NDCs are assigned: by manufacture or distributor, dose, or form. A different color pill results in a different NDC.

Suppression

Even with generalization, you'll probably need some amount of suppression. For the Cajun Code Fest, which had user agreements in place and did not make the data set public, we used an attack simulator to measure average risk using the measure of adversary power explained in "Adversary Power" on page 92. For the level 1 demographic data, we used the same approach we always use for cross-sectional data sets, just like in Chapter 3.

For the level 2 longitudinal data we also used a form of k-anonymity by counting the number of distinct patients in a medical code group, then suppressing codes from the competition data set in which there were fewer than k patients. Notice that we said *distinct* patients—the same patient could have multiple claims with the same medical code, and we don't want to count these more than once. We included the generalized level 1 demographics when we evaluated equivalence classes, though, as well as some level 2 nesting quasi-identifiers that were needed to keep patients within relevant groups.

Picture this: we group patients by their level 1 demographic data, and include the type of place where they received care (e.g., outpatient care, inpatient care, or maybe even a mental health facility). The place of care is a level 2 quasi-identifier and is tied to the claim, but it's at a higher level and is needed to ensure we group patients appropriately based on care. Then we count how many distinct patients have a specific medical code, taking this information into account.

So, a 30- to 39-year-old man (level 1) with an in-hospital (level 2) diagnosis of myocardial infarction (level 2 medical code) who is all alone in this equivalence class will have this medical code suppressed anywhere it appears in his claims.

And we did this for each medical code—Vanderbilt ICD-9 code groups, three-digit CPT codes, and four-character ATC groups—one at a time. That's right, one at a time. Because the risk was low enough, we didn't need to suppress data by considering *k* patients with a particular combination of disease, procedure, and drugs. For the ATC groups we used the dosage form as a nesting variable to ensure that similar drugs were considered together (there's a big difference between a suppository and a pill).

Now, if there's a strong correlation between a disease and a procedure, and one medical code is suppressed because it's not represented by *k* patients, then we expect the other to be suppressed as well. After all, they would have the same nesting variables. But it will depend on how strongly correlated they are, and how many patients have the particular codes. We could treat them as connected variables, but in truth they are different and we don't want to suppress medical codes unless we really have to. Under this scheme, "really have to" means fewer than *k* patients.

We apply this form of longitudinal suppression to every data set we anonymize. You can think of it as a form of strict average risk, which we saw in "Probability Metrics" on page 33, where *k* will be at least two or three distinct patients. Often we'll set *k* to be the inverse of our overall risk threshold. So, if we have a threshold of 0.2, we use $k = 5$; if we have a threshold of 0.1, we use $k = 10$.

We do this to each level 2 field with medical codes individually, linked to the generalized level 1 data and any level 2 quasi-identifier that is of a higher level (e.g., place of service). Obviously, the suppression has to apply to any connected fields as well (such as description fields, or other quasi-identifiers). Suppressing the code for myocardial infarction but not its description would pretty much defeat the purpose of that suppression!

Shuffling

It seems like every day we're shuffling. That's how popular it is with health care users, because they want to maintain the formats of their original fields and end up with realistic-looking data sets. But when it comes to a hackathon, you really want everybody to have a good time—and y'all can't do better than the Cajun Code Fest!

We already mentioned that the organizers gave away the frequencies of the top diseases, procedures, and drugs in a webcast and an online document describing the competition data set. And we've discussed the generalization and suppression we used. But we needed to bring one more trick to the table, so that we could provide the original medical codes, with their original frequencies (bar some suppression to the rarer codes). It just so happens that the trick is something used in pretty much every game of cards.

We start the process off the same way we did for suppression: link all patient claims to their generalized level 1 demographic data. Then we consider all the medical codes in a field that have the same level 1 data plus any level 2 nesting quasi-identifiers. For suppression, we counted all the distinct patients in this set that had the same generalized medical code.

But this time we treat the original codes—within the generalized code group—as a deck of cards, and shuffle them between patients. In other words, we are randomly exchanging exact diagnoses between patients in a code group and their equivalence class. If we didn't do this, then only the code group would be provided in the de-identified data set (since that was the level of generalization deemed suitable through de-identification). You can see that the nesting quasi-identifiers (forming the equivalence class) can be pretty important here. You don't want to swap codes between males and females, or adults and children. The specific codes in a group might also be specific to the place of service, or dosage form, or whatever.

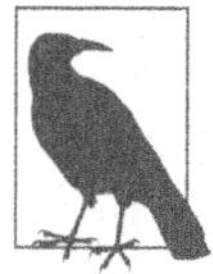

Shuffling is a form of data swapping.[11] The medical code is the swapping attribute—the thing we want to shuffle among similar records—and the demographics and generalized code groups we use to nest the shuffling are called the swapping keys. Statistics on the swapping keys don't change, because they aren't affected by the swapping of medical codes between records. But swapping attributes confuses an adversary that is trying to link records to external information.

The purpose of shuffling is to keep the original codes in the data set, but we want the highest level of data integrity we can get. And of course, we need to use the same nesting quasi-identifiers used in suppression in shuffling. The suppression will ensure we have at least *k* patients in a specific code group and equivalence class, but with shuffling, the adversary can't know which patient in a code group had which original code. That's not to say that shuffling is perfect: though it can create illogical pairings, especially if overly broad code groups are used (e.g., two-digit ICD codes).

Every Day We're Shuffling, But Should You?

If an organization has a data set it needs to de-identify for internal use only, we believe it's acceptable to perform risk mitigation using Vanderbilt ICD-9 code groups and three-digit CPT codes, but leave the original codes in place—no shuffling required. Unknowable pseudonyms need to be used for the patient identifiers, in place of service identifiers though, and any other identifiers that can be tied uniquely to patients.

Also, there need to be restrictions in place against matching your data set to others. When we do a risk assessment with these three-digit codes, we are guarding against attacks based on what a normal person can reasonably know—five-digit ICD codes are too precise for the average person (unless they have another data set to match against). Plus, those three-digit codes already represent hundreds of possible medical categories, which is still very precise for the average person.

Let's say we had four 30- to 39-year-old men with an inpatient diagnosis of ischemic heart disease (Vanderbilt ICD-9 code group 411). Their original diagnoses were intermediate coronary syndrome (411.1), intermediate coronary syndrome again, acute coronary occlusion without myocardial infarction (411.81), and other acute and subacute form of ischemic heart disease (411.89). The original deck therefore had {411.1, 411.1, 411.81, 411.89}, but the shuffled deck had {411.81, 411.1, 411.89, 411.1} (where the position of the code indicates the patient that gets this code, because we're shuffling their diagnoses and not the patients themselves).

For most card games, we can probably get away with a few good riffle shuffles to get good enough randomness. This is how you shuffle a deck of cards in the classic casino scenes of most movies (with half the deck of cards in each hand, the thumbs are lifted so that the cards are interleaved when they are merged into a single deck). In our case we're swapping codes between patients, but it's no different than dealing out a deck of shuffled cards.

But we can do a lot better than "good enough" randomness, given that we have computers at our disposal! Instead, we can program the computer to do the shuffling for us, and be assured that the dealer isn't stacking the deck.

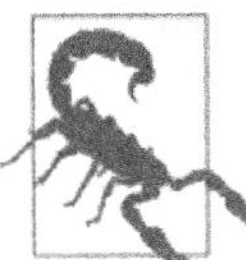

That's not to say that we can use any shuffling algorithm implemented using a computer. Even in a game of cards, top players have been known to take advantage of nonrandomness in a deck. Pseudorandom algorithms in computer randomization also fall into patterns that weaken their effectiveness. What we want is a uniformly distributed random permutation of the rows.

The quick and dirty way to shuffle is to add a column of random numbers, ensuring the probability of getting the same number twice is low, and then sort the rows by ordering them using the column of random numbers. Of course, you want to shuffle within the equivalence class—the level 1 quasi-identifiers and the level 2 nesting quasi-identifiers—so that you can order the rows by the generalized groups and then the random number.

Because the number of codes in each generalized group will be small, you don't need a huge amount of random numbers (remember, you want a low probability of getting the same number twice). A more sophisticated way to permute rows is to use the Fisher-Yates shuffle, which selects a random number from the number of rows being shuffled in its current iteration and then swaps the last row with the random one. But you have to do this within each equivalence class, which would slow down this implementation.

And voilà, you get to keep the original medical codes, with pretty much the same frequencies (barring some suppression in cases where there just aren't enough patients to justify keeping this data, given the risk of re-identification). Perception is reality, and providing medical codes in this way makes the data look like the original!

By shuffling codes, we made it possible to apply all the tools developed at the Cajun Code Fest directly to the original data. The same can be said for testing software, or public data sets and all that can be done with them. Not only is the utility of the data increased (because we can preserve the original frequencies), but people's perception of the data being provided is improved because they can see that it's better data than generalized groups. Even when risk thresholds need to be low, for example in public data sets, shuffling makes the data far more useful and realistic.

Final Thoughts

In a way, we treat medical codes no differently than any other quasi-identifier. To reduce the risk of re-identification, we generalize and suppress. But medical codes are very precise, which means there can be thousands of them. Luckily, some are designed with a logical hierarchy that is easy to take advantage of (e.g., ICD, CPT, and ATC codes), and others we can map to a coding scheme that has the logical hierarchy we need (e.g., NDCs).

And with shuffling we can even go a step further and provide the original codes, not just the generalized groups, with their original frequencies, so that the final de-identified data set has better utility all around. As if the Festival International de Louisiane during Cajun Code Fest wasn't reason enough to dance, this should be.

References

1. Cajun Code Fest (*http://cajuncodefest.org*), "Own Your Own Health."

2. World Health Organization/Centers for Disease Control and Prevention, *International Classification of Diseases*, Ninth Revision, Clinical Modification (ICD-9-CM).

3. American Medical Association, CPT 2012 Professional Edition (*CPT/Current Procedural Terminology (Professional Edition)*) (Chicago, IL: AMA Press, 2011).

4. K. El Emam, D. Paton, F. Dankar, and G. Koru, "De-Identifying a Public Use Microdata File from the Canadian National Discharge Abstract Database," *BMC Medical Informatics and Decision Making* 11:(2011): 53

5. J.C. Denny, M.D. Ritchie, M. Basford, J. Pulley, L. Bastarache, K. Brown-Gentry, D. Wang, D.R. Masys, D.M. Roden, and D.C. Crawford, "PheWAS: Demonstrating the Feasibility of a Phenome-Wide Scan to Discover Gene–Disease Associations," *Bioinformatics* 26:9 (2010): 1205–1210.

6. A. Elixhauser, C. Steiner, and L. Palmer, *Clinical Classifications Software (CCS)* (*http://1.usa.gov/ccs-guide*) (US Agency for Healthcare Research and Quality), 2011.

7. G.J. Escobar, J.D. Greene, P. Scheirer, M.N. Gardner, D. Draper, and P. Kipnis. "Risk-Adjusting Hospital Inpatient Mortality Using Automated Inpatient, Outpatient, and Laboratory Databases," *Medical Care* 46:(2008): 232–9.

8. K. El Emam, L. Arbuckle, G. Koru, B. Eze, L. Gaudette, E. Neri, S. Rose, J. Howard, and J. Gluck, "De-Identification Methods for Open Health Data: The Case of the Heritage Health Prize Claims Dataset," *Journal of Medical Internet Research* 14:1(2012): e33.

9. WHO Collaborating Centre for Drug Statistics Methodology "Guidelines for ATC classification and DDD assignment 2011 (*http://bit.ly/whocc-guide*)," (Oslo, 2010).

10. N.C. Santanello and E. Bortnichak, "Creation of Standardized Coding Libraries—A Call to Arms for Pharmacoepidemiologists," *PharmacoEpi and Risk Management Newsletter* 2:(2009): 6–7.

11. G.T. Duncan, M. Elliot, and J.-J. Salazar-González, *Statistical Confidentiality* (New York: Springer. 2011.)

CHAPTER 11

Masking: Oncology Databases

When we need to remove all useful data from a field, we turn to data masking—the second of our pillars discussed in "The Two Pillars of Anonymization" on page 5. Usually this means replacing real data with entirely random values, possibly from a large database (for things like names). Obviously, this isn't something we do to fields we need for analytics. Rather, it's something we apply to things like names, Social Security numbers, and ID fields. De-identification involves protecting fields we need for analytics, and is a trade-off between privacy and utility; masking involves protecting fields we don't need for analytics, and is meant to completely hide the original data.

To understand the reasons for masking and its trade-offs, we'll take a short look at a real database. The American Society of Clinical Oncology (ASCO) (*http://www.asco.org*) has launched an ambitious project to build tools on top of oncology electronic health record (EHR) data collected from sites across the country. Its goal is to improve the quality of care by having millions of patients essentially participate in a large clinical trial, pooling all of their data in a system called CancerLinQ.[1]

Schema Shmema

Before we discuss data masking, let's look at an example database that the ASCO CancerLinQ system may come across. This will give us examples to think about when we go through approaches to masking. Figure 11-1 is a schema for our invented database. Direct identifiers include the names, address (although we'll keep the ZIP code as a quasi-identifier), and SSN. But the patient ID is unique to the patient, at least within the EHR, so it also has to be masked (better safe than sorry). Short free-form text fields might contain identifying information, like the patient's name, so unless we're going to de-identify that we'll need to mask it as well.

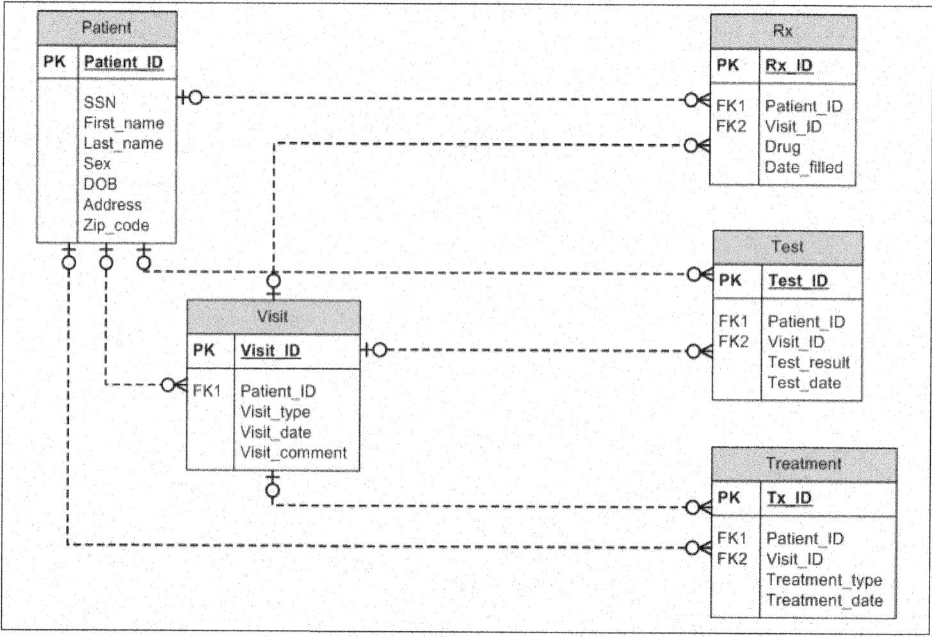

Figure 11-1. Like a school of herring, these tables stick together. Of course, this is only one example schema for an oncology database; there could be many variations.

Data in Disguise

The term "data masking" is used mostly in industry, and it packages the techniques that are applied to deal with direct identifiers. There are three defensible approaches to data masking. If implemented properly, they will ensure that the risk of re-identification is extremely small. And because these approaches will, by definition, ensure small risk, it's not necessary to evaluate risk levels for masking. Just implementing the recommended masking schemes is sufficient.

Field Suppression

Suppression is by far the simplest way to mask data—just remove the direct identifiers from the data set. This could be done with the first name, last name, and SSN, to name a few. It's perfect for those pesky comment fields we mentioned in the oncology database, since we don't know what's in them and really, since they're just short notes, we don't need them. If we did, we would turn to the methods to anonymize free-form text that we discussed in Chapter 8.

Suppression is an acceptable approach in some situations. If we're disclosing a data set to a researcher, it's pretty unlikely that he'll need any of these fields. An exception would be if the researcher were planning to contact the patients; then having their names would help. But then it wouldn't be an anonymized data set.

Another situation that often comes up is when the researcher wants to link the data set with another one, so the SSN is needed for the purpose of linking. But we don't want to disclose SSN values in the clear because it's personal information. We'll see how to get around this in Chapter 12, where we describe a method for linking on unique identifiers, such as the SSN, without revealing the actual values to the researcher.

But suppression isn't always acceptable. When developing health applications, there's a need to test software. It's necessary to work with realistic data to perform meaningful functional and performance testing of applications. The most realistic data is real data, coming from live production systems. But you do not want to give your development teams real patient data.

Software testing would definitely be considered a secondary use of the data. This raises all of the usual regulatory issues around using identifiable data for secondary purposes without consent. But there are also known, and well-publicized, cases of the development team losing patient data.[2]

When testing a software application, it's necessary to maintain all of the fields in that database in their original format. You can't suppress entire fields because the data must fill in all of the database columns to facilitate testing. Field suppression is simply not an option here.

A related example is when users of health applications run into problems with the software, possibly due to bugs. They'll want to send you some sample data to recreate the problem, so that your development team can fix it quickly. You would want to mask any identifying data before sending it to the development team, but you wouldn't want to suppress identifying fields in case they're causing the problem. Similar examples include use for software demos and training.

Randomization

Randomization is the process of replacing the direct identifier values with fake data: fake person names, for example, or fake SSNs. The fake values can be generated independently of the data, using random characters for names and random numbers for SSNs. Or the fake values can be selected randomly from a large database of known values, such as a database of real first names and last names. Randomization can result in some very real-looking data sets.

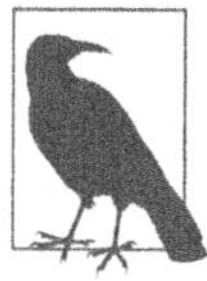

If values are being selected from a database, the database should be large enough to render the probability of selecting any one name very small. Randomization can also be performed to enforce uniqueness: for example, replace every name with a unique name. We definitely need to enforce uniqueness when randomizing patient and facility IDs in the oncology database; otherwise, relationships in the data will be lost.

Some conditions can be placed on the randomization. A perfect example is tying names to the patient's sex, so that patients are assigned more or less sex-specific names. It would make sense to use typically female names for breast cancer data, or typically male names for prostate cancer data. But you have to be careful about how specific the conditions should be. You don't want to give away information, so the conditions that you match to should be in the de-identified data. If you've dropped the patient's sex from the data set, forget about matching name to sex. Otherwise, the name would leak information about the patient's sex.

Replacing names with random names that have the same length would also be a bad idea (due to the possibility of a frequency attack). Some surnames have 20 characters, but only a handful, and maybe only in a particular geography. If an adversary can know the length of the name, she might be able to figure out the original name. And it's extremely unlikely that the length of a person's name is otherwise included in the data set. (If so, then include it as a quasi-identifier, although we've never heard of such a thing!)

We looked at the North Carolina voter registration list, which is available publicly, and found that there were only two people with first names having 17 characters, four people with last names having 16 characters, and three people with last names having 21 characters. We also looked at a registry of lawyers and doctors in Ontario, and there was only person with a first name having 17, 18, or 20 characters, and only one person with a last name having 24 characters.

It's possible to include ethnicity in a de-identified data set, so this could be used as a condition on which names are randomized. For example, if there's a field indicating that a patient is Asian, then an Asian name would be used in the randomization. But otherwise, it's a bad idea to use this strategy to randomize names, as it will inadvertently increase the risk of re-identification.

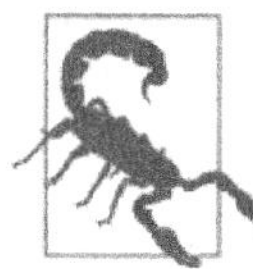

When you use both masking and de-identification on a data set, any masking that depends on a quasi-identifier needs to be applied after de-identification. So, if the first name is being randomized on the condition of the patient's sex, make sure you do the masking on the de-identified sex field so that suppression is taken into account. Otherwise, you might leak the sex of the patient where you had intended to have it removed!

When randomizing fields in a relational database, ensuring consistency is important. The schema in Figure 11-1 is normalized, so the names do not appear in multiple tables. But there are many databases out there that are not normalized—e.g., the *First_name* and *Last_name* fields might appear in other tables as well. If the *Last_name* is randomized to "Herring" from "Salmon," then all instances of *Last_name* for that patient in other tables will also be converted to "Herring."

Pseudonymization

Pseudonymization replaces one or more direct identifiers with some other unique value. It is also called coding, single coding, double coding, masking, obfuscation, and tokenization. They all in essence mean the same thing.

For example, an SSN may be replaced with another fake SSN value. We consider pseudonyms to be derived from the original value. Therefore, if we have an SSN and we generate a pseudonym from it repeatedly, we will always get the same pseudonym value. This is an important characteristic of pseudonyms because it allows the matching of patient records across time.

Suppose we have a database of patients that we're using for testing and we create pseudonyms from their SSNs. Then, after six months, we get an update to that database. Because the pseudonym generated for each patient will be the same in the original database and the new increment, it will be possible to determine which records belong to the same patient.

Two general methods are used to generate pseudonyms: hashing and encryption. With hashing it's necessary to add a random value called a *salt* to the SSN to foil dictionary attacks on the pseudonym. This salt must not be shared with any outsider, because it's essentially a key to unlock the pseudonym.

The disadvantage of hashing is that it results in a large value: 32, 44, or 64 bytes when converted to an ASCII string. If our database has allocated 11 characters for an SSN field, we won't be able to stuff the hash of that SSN into the field. Recall also that in some situations, such as software testing, we want to maintain the integrity of the database, which includes all of the fields and their types.

Format-preserving encryption is a type of encryption that will create an encrypted value that can fit into the same field length as the original value. It also uses a secret key that must be kept in a safe place. It solves the problem of ensuring that the database schema is not distorted after the pseudonym is created.

Referential integrity is also an important capability for pseudonyms, because these pseudonyms are often used to link individuals' records across tables. This can be maintained in the same manner as for randomization schemes. If an identifier is converted to a pseudonym in one table, then it will need to be converted in the same manner in all tables in the database. In our schema in Figure 11-1, the *Patient_ID* might be converted to a pseudonym in the *Patient* table. But to ensure that the tables can be joined properly, that same *Patient_ID* would need to be converted to the same pseudonym in other tables, such as the *Visit* table or the *Rx* table.

Controlled Re-Identification

In some cases it's necessary to determine the identity of the data subject. For example, in a public health context it may be determined that an individual has been exposed to a substance or pathogen that requires follow-up, or that contact tracing is required. In those cases it may be necessary to reverse the pseudonyms created.

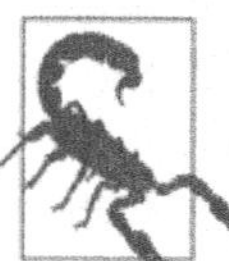

Reversing pseudonyms needs to be performed in a secure environment, with appropriate controls and oversight, and under conditions that have been defined in advance (not willy-nilly, when the mood arises). You need to be sure that the re-identification of individuals is legitimate.

To allow the reversing of pseudonyms that are hash values, you need to maintain a mapping table between the pseudonyms and the original values. This mapping table needs to be kept in a secure place and referred to only when a re-identification is necessary.

When you have used format-preserving encryption, the only thing you need to store securely is the encryption key. The key can then be used to decrypt the pseudonym and recover the original values. The advantage here is that a whole mapping table doesn't need to be kept. For large data sets, this mapping table can grow significantly in size.

Frequency of Pseudonyms

We have to be careful with pseudonyms, as they could still leak information through their frequency. If unique identifiers, such as MRNs or SSNs, are converted to pseudonyms using the methods we describe, then there shouldn't be leakage of information.

However, sometimes pseudonyms are created for other types of fields, such as facility names or even regions.

Consider a data set where there's a field indicating the hospital where care was provided. As part of data masking the hospital name was converted to a pseudonym. This conversion seems to hide the hospital name, but allows an analyst to know which patients went to the same hospital. So far, so good.

Now, in the city we live in, Ottawa, there's one very large hospital and a few small hospitals. Most adult patients go The Ottawa Hospital (TOH). Any data set of patients discharged from Ottawa hospitals will have a high frequency for the pseudonym of TOH. It doesn't matter what the pseudonym is; its frequency will make it obvious which pseudonym is for TOH. Similarly, there's only one children's hospital in the region, and the hospital pseudonym that has the highest frequency of pediatric discharges will most likely be for the children's hospital.

An adversary can therefore reverse engineer the hospital using only frequency information. Performing a test to determine if the pseudonym distribution deviates too much from a uniform distribution should reveal these types of situations.

A better approach is to dichotomize that field into "TOH Patients" and "Non-TOH Patients," then include that new dichotomous field in the usual re-identification risk assessment (effectively treating it as a quasi-identifier). If a particular value is suppressed, then that pseudonym is also suppressed. If a value in the new dichotomous field is not suppressed, then it's OK to reveal that pseudonym. The nesting can be more complex, though.

This isn't just for hospitals—there are specialty centers in Ottawa as well (there's a heart institute, a cancer center, and an eye institute). So, these concerns apply to the frequencies within a particular diagnosis group as well.

Masking On the Fly

Masking functionality can be embedded between the database and the presentation layer of an application. The presentation layer may be a summary table from a data set, or a data export. When the data from the database is pulled out to be processed, the fields that are designated as direct identifiers are then masked automatically and the masked values are transmitted on to the next layer in the application.

On-the-fly masking is being considered for the CancerLinQ system that ASCO is developing, depending on user access privileges. It's currently still in the prototype phase, so this is not implemented, but it would certainly help give different users different layers of access.

Generally, this kind of approach works well in environments where the data is dynamic, changing on a regular basis. It's also suitable when the database scheme is fixed and the direct identifiers can be determined in advance. Data users are assured that any data extracted from the database is always masked. The automated masking eliminates the need for manual interventions to ensure that the data is properly masked.

Of course, the setup for on-the-fly masking would need to be updated every time the database scheme was changed (for example, if a new direct identifier was added to the database).

Final Thoughts

It should be clear in reading this book that masking alone is not nearly enough to protect the identity of an individual. Masking is necessary, but it's not sufficient. The other methods that we've presented for de-identification must also be used. The reason we reiterate this point is that we still see organizations that are handling sensitive health information who do only masking without de-identification. These organizations are taking a nontrivial risk, but if you're reading this book, you know better.

References

1. R. Winslow, " 'Big Data' for Cancer Care: Vast Storehouse of Patient Records Will Let Doctors Search for Effective Treatment," *The Wall Street Journal*, 27 March 2013.

2. S. Rubenstein, "Express Scripts Data Breach Leads to Extortion Attempt," *The Wall Street Journal*, 7 November 2008.

CHAPTER 12

Secure Linking

A lot of useful health data is *linked* health data. This means that the data set consists of multiple data sets that have been linked together. But anonymization, by design, makes linking difficult. How do you accurately link records together between two data sets when they have next to nothing in common after anonymization? This is a challenge we see a lot with anonymization. Data sets are collected at different points in time, or by different organizations, and they need to be linked together to run the desired analytics.

To be useful for analysis, data sets must be linked *before* anonymization. This means that the different organizations holding the constituent data sets need to share information to allow this linking to happen. The best fields to use for linking data sets are almost always identifiers, which means that the organizations have to share personally identifying information in order to link their data. We're back to the original problem now—how can these organizations share personal identifiers if they do not have appropriate authority or consent?

Only once they're linked can the data sets be de-identified and used and disclosed for secondary purposes. We've seen many useful projects die because it wasn't possible to link the needed data sets together. But this problem can be solved: this chapter describes a way to securely link data sets together without disclosing personal information. The mechanism is an equi-join process for two tables that have one or more common fields that act as unique identifiers.

Let's Link Up

There are many situations where linking health data sets is necessary or can help facilitate powerful analytics. For instance, clinical data from electronic medical records at a family practice could be linked to hospital discharge data and retail pharmacy data. This linked data would show how treatment by a primary care physician after patients have been discharged from the hospital can affect complications from their hospital procedures. It provides a more complete picture of the continuum of care that patients experience.

Emergency department visits can be mapped to prescription or dispensation of drugs to evaluate drug side effects or interactions. Data on vital statistics could also be added to include deaths, to evaluate survival rates for different paths through the health care system, or to compare treatments. These are straightforward data linking cases, but they require a way to uniquely identify individuals between the data sets.

The data sets that need to be linked do not necessarily have to come from the providers. Researchers may have survey data on the sexual behaviors of youths, and it may be valuable to link that data with HPV vaccination information to determine whether the highest-risk individuals are being vaccinated. That means matching records from a research data set with a vaccination registry. Securing such sensitive health information is obviously a high priority.

Figuring out when patients have died for a survival analysis could also use the National Death Index (NDI). The way this usually works is that researchers submit their records to the NDI, which then performs the matching for them and sends back information about the matching records. The data being sent to the NDI could be just about anything, such as a list of patients diagnosed with cancer, or those on some specific diet, or nothing whatsoever (for a baseline).

Health data can also be linked with nonhealth data. Immigration data can be linked to health insurance claims data to examine how new immigrants' health evolves when they settle in their adoptive countries. Correctional services data can be linked with health data to examine the health of inmates after they return to the community. And educational data can be linked with health data to determine the impact of infant health on school performance.

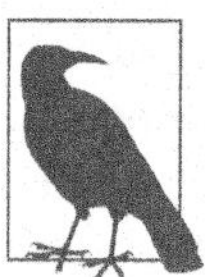

As the previous examples illustrate, often different parties will own the individual databases that we need to link together. Some of them will be health care providers, and some will have nothing to do with health care but still hold valuable data. Anonymization methods could be applied before the data is shared among all of these different parties. The anonymization would ensure that the risk of re-identifying the data subjects is very small, and would eliminate some key barriers to these organizations sharing their data. But it would also make it very challenging for them to link their data together!

Secure methods for linking two databases can also address two other very common use cases: secure lookup and de-duplication.

Secure lookup is the use case where we want to find whether a record in one table exists in the other table without revealing identifying information about the record. For instance, imagine two parties, the Carolers and the Tailgaters, that each have a table. The Tailgaters have a record about "Billy" in their table, and they want to find out whether Billy is in the table that the Carolers are holding. However, they do not want to reveal the identity of Billy to the Carolers, and they do not even want the Carolers to know whether the record was found in the Tailgaters' table. Nor do the Carolers want to share their table with the Tailgaters, because they don't want the Tailgaters to learn the identities of the other individuals in the Carolers' table. At the end of the secure lookup, the only information revealed to the Tailgaters is whether Billy is in the Carolers' table. This scenario is exactly the same as secure linking, except that the linking is performed on a single record.

Secure lookups are useful in fraud detection. For example, let's say an insurance company has received a claim for some procedure that Billy has undergone, but they are suspicious and want to see whether the same claim was also submitted to one of their competitors. Billy and his provider may be completely innocent, so it would be inappropriate to reveal their identities until there is evidence to warrant further investigation. Also, the competing insurance company does not want to reveal its client database. A secure lookup would allow the first insurance company to do a lookup in the second company's database without revealing the identity of the individual being sought, and without knowing who else is in that second company's database.

Also consider a government department that provides health insurance to low-income individuals, and that wants to confirm that insurance recipients indeed have a low income. The tax department has all of the data on income. However, the health department is not allowed to share information with the tax department, and vice versa. A secure lookup would allow the health department to know whether Billy, who is receiving insurance, is indeed claiming a low income, without revealing Billy's identity to the tax department and without getting access to the tax information of the rest of the population.

The second use case is *de-duplication*, which means removing duplicate entries. Here, two complete tables are linked, but just for the purpose of de-duplicating records. De-duplication is a critical step in producing data sets that are clean and ready for analytical use. For example, all states collect uniform data for cancer surveillance on people diagnosed and treated while living in their jurisdiction. They count those cases to calculate statewide cancer incidence rates. The state of residence at the time of diagnosis and treatment is a crucial piece of information to determine population-based cancer incidence. Each state works independently to identify cases. What they don't want is to count patients that reside in multiple jurisdictions more than once, perhaps because they have a summer home or cottage (like those lucky "snowbirds"). So, they need to de-duplicate their registries, but without sharing the identities of individuals who reside in only a single state. A secure linking protocol would allow this to be accomplished.

Doing It Securely

The tables held by the Carolers and the Tailgaters have some fields in common. The tables also have the same or overlapping patients. We need to join these two tables using a unique identifier for individuals. The unique identifier might be a Social Security number, a health card insurance number, a medical record number, or a credit card number. It can also be a combination of variables that are uniquely identifying, such as county of birth, date of birth, gender, first initial, and last name.

But these unique identifiers are sensitive pieces of information, and it's often quite challenging to share them among organizations. In Ontario, if a researcher wants to collect the health insurance number for the purpose of linking the records of research subjects, he will need to get approval from his ethics board. Most ethics boards would be reluctant to grant that approval, which means that if a researcher needs to link two databases the health insurance number may not be used, even though it's the best unique identifier for all citizens.

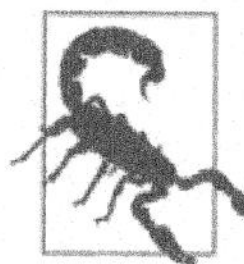

Although we're just looking to link records in the data, sometimes these unique identifiers can themselves be used to identify an individual. For example, you might think Social Security numbers are simply random numbers assigned to people for the purpose of managing information about them. But it's possible to figure out a person's identity from this number,[1] making its use equivalent to sharing personal identifiable information. That's not to mention that Social Security numbers are so widely collected that they can be used to identify people from other data sources.

It would be nice if one party could just give its data to the other one and have that party join the two tables together. The linked data set could then be de-identified and used or disclosed for secondary purposes. But in a lot of cases that's just not going to happen, and rightly so, because of privacy concerns for those patients who aren't in both tables. Parties often don't even have the authority to share identifying information about their patients. What we need is a way to allow this linking without sharing identifying fields. For this we turn to encryption, which means protecting data inside of an encoding scheme that doesn't allow anyone to understand what it is without a key.

Don't Try This at Home

A number of methods have been used in the past to link data sets together, but they're either not very secure or quite expensive. We'll describe these here so you know what not to do. Assume that the Carolers want to de-duplicate their data against the data from the Tailgaters by matching on the health card number (HCN). Here are some of the possibilities:

Matching on hashed values

A simple scheme is for the Carolers and Tailgaters to hash their HCNs (basically creating a map from a key to a value, to mask the information and speed up comparisons). The Carolers would send their hashed values to the Tailgaters. The Tailgaters would then match the hashed values to figure out how many and which ones are duplicates. The problem with this approach is that the Tailgaters can hash all possible HCNs and compare these with what they get from the Carolers. If the HCN consists of nine digits, the Tailgaters would need to generate only one billion hashed values, and use these as a dictionary (from hash to HCN). The Tailgaters could then reverse engineer the HCNs for all of the data they received. Not so secure. Don't do this.

Matching on hashed values with a third party

The Carolers and the Tailgaters could each send their hashed values to a trusted third party, the Easter Bunnies (and who doesn't trust the Easter Bunnies?). The Easter Bunnies would then match the hashed values and return the result to the Carolers. This would allow them to de-duplicate their database, yay! Oh, wait, the Easter Bunnies could easily launch the same dictionary attack on both sets of hashed values to reverse engineer the original values. We're willing to trust the Easter Bunnies, but not that much. (Otherwise, what was the point of using hashed values in the first place?)

Salting the hash

It's possible for the Tailgaters and the Carolers to add a random value to the HCNs before hashing them. Such salting of the hash is often attempted as a way to protect against the flaws already noted. But because the salt value needs to be shared with both parties, either one can still launch a dictionary attack on the data. We're back to square one, with the same basic problem as before.

Salting the hash with a third party

Now, if both the Carolers and the Tailgaters salt their hashes with the same random value independently of one another, and send the results to the Easter Bunnies, the Easter Bunnies can do the matching and we avoid the dictionary attack problem. The Easter Bunnies don't know the salt value—right? Well, not quite. This approach requires the Carolers and the Tailgaters to share a secret, their salt value, with each other. Sharing secrets is generally not recommended because if either of them loses or discloses the salt, they essentially compromise the security of the other's data.

Those of you working in the security space will be thinking, "No way, this doesn't happen." Oh, but it does. We've seen it. Security protocols are detailed and nuanced. Not everyone will appreciate, and therefore follow, all the steps down to the letter, or understand their limitations. They'll do what they think is secure, but it often isn't. We call this practicing security without a license.

The Third-Party Problem

You might think that there can't possibly be too many parties (birthday parties, tailgate parties, Easter parties). But, alas, that simply isn't the case here. A general challenge with approaches that require a trusted third party is that when the Carolers and Tailgaters are in different jurisdictions, they may not agree on who that third party will be. Each one of them will want the third party to be in their jurisdiction because they don't quite trust parties in other jurisdictions. This makes protocols using a trusted third party difficult to implement.

Creating a trusted third party is also expensive, because a lot of security and privacy practices and protocols need to be in place. The third party also needs to be audited on a regular basis to ensure compliance with the stipulated practices and protocols. The Carolers and Tailgaters may agree to trust the Easter Bunnies as their secure third party, but it's also a lot of overhead for the Easter Bunnies to take on.

The Three Shades of Parties

There are generally three kinds of parties that participate in security protocols:

Fully trusted parties
: We let these parties go their own way. We trust them not to get out of hand. They get access to personal information, and we know full well they would be able to easily attack the information they get to recover personal information, but we trust them not to do so. But as we've noted already, this assumption has some inherent disadvantages.

Semi-trusted parties
: OK, so we can't all be that trusting. Instead, we trust with caveats. We assume that each party will follow the protocol as specified, but recognize that they could use the information they receive and the output of their computations to recover personal information. For example, if you give the Birthdaygoers a piece of software to run, they'll execute it as expected, but they might intercept the inputs and outputs to the software and then use that information in some way.

Malicious parties
: These are the ones we have to watch out for. Let's call them the Ravers. They may not follow the protocol, and they may deliberately deviate from the protocol to recover personal information. They could, as a deliberate deviation, be injecting fake values into the output.

In protocols developed in the context of health care, we assume that we're dealing with semi-trusted parties.

Some protocols that are used quite extensively in practice for linking health data use a *fourth* trusted party. The fourth party generates the salt value and embeds it within a software program. In our example, the Carolers and Tailgaters then execute that software program to hash the values, and then send the hashed values to their trusted third party, the Easter Bunnies, to link them. This approach would be secure if we assumed that the Carolers and Tailgaters would not, or cannot, reverse engineer the software program to attempt to recover the salt value.

The challenge with using a fourth trusted party is that it amplifies the complexity of the linking protocol and amplifies the disadvantages of having a trusted third party. Plus, what are we going to call this fourth party? We're running out of amusing names!

Basic Layout for Linking Up

We start with our two parties, the Carolers and the Tailgaters, that want to join their databases together. The Carolers have a database with a bunch of records; the Tailgaters have a database with another bunch of records. Of course, they need a set of fields in common on which to match the databases together.

We need to consider a few points in devising this kind of equi-join protocol:

- One of the two parties, probably the Carolers, might not have much in the way of computing power. They have data, and they're willing to provide it, but they don't want to invest in anything other than what they already have to help with the secure equi-join. This is just a practical requirement because often one entity wants to link or de-duplicate against another larger entity's database. The former will not have much computing capacity and does not want to invest in developing that capacity because it does not need to do the linking very often. This requirement necessitates that we have some kind of third party involved in the protocol.
- It should be possible for only one party, the Carolers, to know the results of the match. The Carolers might be checking the data in the NDI for their cancer survival analysis. But they don't want the Tailgaters, who work at the NDI, to know which patients they're looking for.
- Because of the disadvantages of having trusted third parties, discussed in "The Third-Party Problem" on page 176, it's best to avoid using them if possible. Where they do exist, such as in the case of national statistical agencies, they probably don't have the mandate to act as third parties anyway.
- A semi-trusted third party, the Birthdaygoers, would work, though. They're trusted to follow the protocol, but nothing more. They might be a little too eager to try and discover PHI, which is why they aren't fully trusted. But that's OK, because they won't be given any info that would allow them to discover PHI, so strong security measures don't need to be put in place for what they handle.

- Neither the Carolers nor Tailgaters needs to share secrets. They keep to themselves, so that no one party needs to trust the other. Otherwise, if the Tailgaters lost the shared key, the encrypted or hashed data of the Carolers would also be jeopardized, and they would be singing a new tune.
- The matching between individuals in the two databases needs to be unique for the equi-join to work. The matching variables could include unique individual identifiers, or combinations of identifiers that together are unique, such as names and dates of birth.
- The Tailgaters are assumed to have significant computing power. They will do much of the heavy lifting. This makes sense because the Tailgaters are the ones with the valuable data resource that everyone wants to link to. This makes it economical for them to invest in some computing capacity.

Ultimately, the architecture of the equi-join protocol requires a semi-trusted third party, the Birthdaygoers. The Birthdaygoers act as the key holder. The key holder needs to have decent computing resources, but it won't learn the identities of the patients or learn anything new about them during the process of the equi-join. The only thing that the Birthdaygoers will learn within this protocol is how many patients matched between the two data sets.

The Nitty-Gritty Protocol for Linking Up

Unfortunately, we need to get our hands dirty and dig into some technical details to make linked data work. The basic idea is that we'll use encryption to hide the inner workings of the equi-join.

Bringing Paillier to the Parties

Let's look at the additive homomorphic encryption system proposed by Paillier.[2,3] Wow, that's already a mouthful. *Additive* means exactly what you think, except that we're adding encrypted data, which is kind of cool when you think about it. Take two encrypted pieces of information, add them together, and you get their sum. Except it's still encrypted, so you have no idea what that sum is! *Homomorphism* is basically a map that preserves the structure between two sets that have some predefined operations performed on them—operations that take in a finite number of elements to produce an output. OK, so what we have, more or less, is an encryption system that allows addition with operators that can take a finite set of elements to produce an output. So far, so good.

With the Paillier cryptosystem it's possible to perform mathematical operations on the encrypted values themselves, notably addition and limited forms of multiplication. We start by picking two really big prime numbers at random, then we multiply them to give us a value p. Let's consider two data elements, m_1 and m_2, and their encrypted values, $E(m_1)$ and $E(m_2)$:

Paillier addition

$E(m_1) \times E(m_2) = E(m_1 + m_2)$, where multiplication of cyphertext is mod p^2 and addition of plaintext is mod p in this algebraic system

Decrypting this information gives us $D(E(m_1 + m_2)) = m_1 + m_2$. So, this cryptosystem is mapping multiplication of cyphertext (the encrypted values) to addition of plaintext (the unencrypted values). Pretty cool, but let's not forget that the encryption and decryption require a key:

Paillier multiplication

$(E(m_1))^{m_2} = E(m_1 \times m_2)$, where exponentiation of cyphertext is mod p^2 and multiplication of plaintext is mod p

Decrypting this information gives us $D(E(m_1 \times m_2)) = m_1 \times m_2$. This time the value m_2 is plaintext only, not encrypted. The value m_1 is encrypted, and the product of m_1 and m_2 is encrypted, but not m_2 itself. That's what makes this a limited form of multiplication. Unfortunately, there isn't a way to do multiplication of cyphertext in this system.

An important property of Paillier encryption is that it's probabilistic: it uses randomness in its encryption algorithm so that encrypting the same message several times will generally give different cyphertexts. This ensures that an adversary won't be able to compare encrypted messages to figure out the underlying information.

Matching on the Unknown

First things first. The Birthdaygoers need to generate a key pair—a public encryption key and a private decryption key—and send the public key to the Tailgaters and the Carolers, as shown in Figure 12-1. What we want to do is match on the unknown, i.e., the encrypted values.

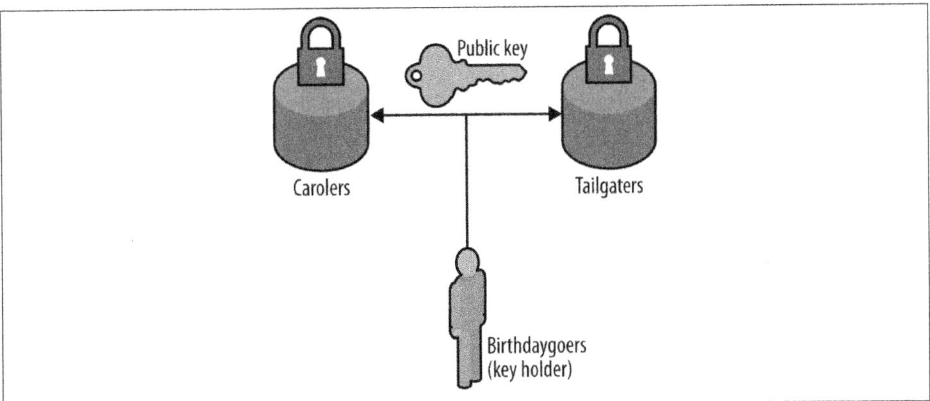

Figure 12-1. The first step in any relationship is to share (in this case, the public encryption key).

The Carolers initiate the matching (they're very responsible that way, going door to door bringing cheer). For nonstring fields (e.g., SSN or HCN), we use a secure comparison to find matches between records in the data set sent by the Carolers and what the Tailgaters already have. This works as shown in Figure 12-2, and is described in more detail in the following list:

1. The Carolers send their encrypted records to the Tailgaters (which will be used in a couple of steps). Let *E(x)* be one of their encrypted HCNs. Obviously they need to send all of them, but we want to use minimal notation for simplicity.
2. For each encrypted record the Tailgaters have, *E(y)*, they generate a random number *r* to accompany it. Each record gets a new random number (no double dipping!).
3. For every pair of records between the Carolers and the Tailgaters, and over every matching variable, they compute the funky comparison variable $c = ((E(x) \times E(y))^{-1})^r$. So, it's one funky comparison variable for each pair of records, and each matching variable. Recall that every matching variable, which is then sent to the Birthdaygoers, has its own encryption.
4. The Birthdaygoers use their private key to decrypt the *c* values, and blow party horns when these values equal zero! Because a zero means a match, which sounds like a good enough reason to blow a party horn when you're a Birthdaygoer. Non-zero values mean that there isn't a match, so no party horns.
5. The Birthdaygoers are left with a binary table of matches and nonmatches, basically a bingo card, for all of the compared pairs of records and matching variables. The final bingo card of matches can be sent back to whoever it is that's planning to link the two data sets together.

Although that description was for nonstring fields, the basic idea works equally well for string fields. The major difference is that you need to consider the approximate matching of strings, in case there are first or last names that have typos or some other difference. Phonetic encoding functions, like Soundex and NYSIIS, can be used to perform exact comparisons in the same way we showed before.

We can even match records on approximate birth dates, following the guidelines used by the NDI. We consider records matched on dates of birth when any of the following are found in the two records:

- Exact same month and same year of birth
- Exact same month and same day of birth
- Exact same month and year of birth to within one year

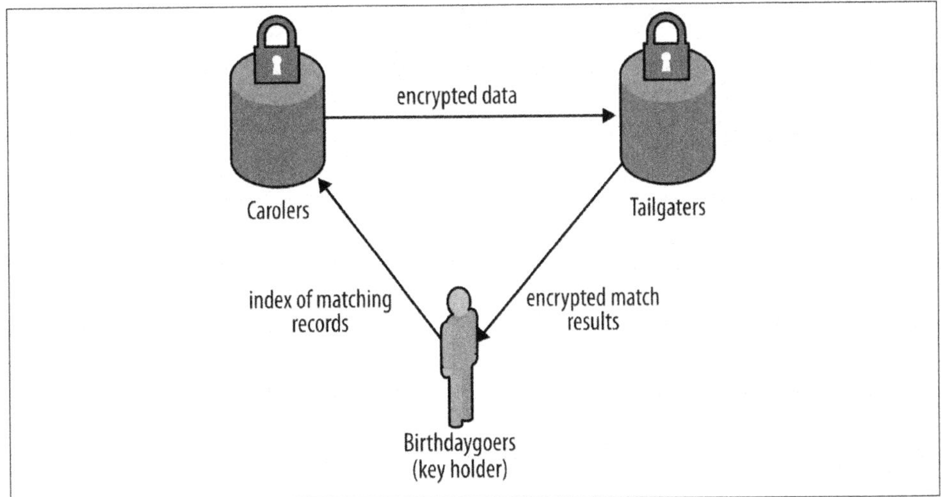

Figure 12-2. Now we share data for the matching of records.

For the matching protocol this means we would need to share the encrypted values for the day, month, year – 1, year, and year + 1 of the date of birth (i.e., five different encrypted values). And be careful of differences in the order of day, month, and year when comparing dates! One database might use day/month/year, and another month/day/year.

Scaling Up

The protocol we just described will, sadly, not scale very well. If the Carolers have a database with n records, and the Tailgaters have a database with m records, we will need to do $n \times m$ comparisons. This can be a pretty big number for large databases, and all of these comparisons can take a long time—computations on encrypted values are slower than computations on raw (unencrypted) values. We need to make the protocol run more efficiently than that.

One approach is to use *blocking*, where we do some data partitioning up front. Let's take our example of matching on the HCNs. The Carolers send along the year of birth as well as the encrypted HCN. (For it to be safe for them to send this information, the year of birth for the data held by the Carolers would have to have a low risk of re-identification, as measured using the techniques described earlier in this book.) If there are 50 unique years of birth in the data set and they are uniformly distributed, we have essentially split the data set into 50 mini data sets. No HCN can match any HCN associated with a different year of birth, so the number of comparisons required could be 50 times fewer in this case.

If this is not enough, we can add another variable to block on; let's say the state. If there are 50 states in the data set, the combination of state and year of birth could result in as many as 2,500 unique values. Then we would end up with 2,500 fewer comparisons. Now we're cookin'!

Of course, we would have to be sure that the combination of year of birth and state has a low risk of re-identification for the Carolers' data set.

These are nontrivial performance improvements, but we can still do better.

Cuckoo Hashing

Cuckoo hashing is a well-developed hashing scheme about which you can find many technical articles. This isn't necessarily an easy concept to grasp, but we'll try to explain without going into too much detail. To describe it in the context of our linking problem, the Carolers would create a hash table to store their encrypted HCN values. The hash table would have a "bin" for each encrypted value. This hash table would allow the Tailgaters to find the right bins when doing their comparisons.

For each HCN, the Carolers would compute the index for its bin and store its value in that bin. When all of the HCNs have been inserted in the hash table, any empty bins are filled up with fake encrypted values. That way, the frequency of the HCNs is not disclosed. This meets one of the goals of cryptography, which is to share as little information as possible. It's crazy what can be used to attack encrypted data if there's any leakage of information—even the time it takes to execute a protocol can be used to attack the system. Better to not have any leakage.

This padded hash table is sent to the Tailgaters. They take each one of their own HCN numbers and compute its bin index. Then they pull the value in that bin from the hash table they received from the Carolers, and compare the values. An interesting feature of a cuckoo hash table is that the Tailgaters need to look in only two bins to know with a high probability whether there's a match or not. This means that the total number of comparisons will be $2 \times m$, irrespective of how large the Carolers' table is (which has n records). That is cuckoo, but good cuckoo.

How Fast Does a Cuckoo Run?

To illustrate how fast this can run in practice, we did a few evaluations on a series of HCNs of various sizes The results are shown in Table 12-1. Here, the tables for the Carolers and Tailgaters were of the same size. We used a 64-bit Windows 2008 server machine with eight cores.

Table 12-1. Cuckoo hashing performance

No. of records (each)	Encryption (secs)	Compare (secs)	Match (secs)	Total time
10,000	16	29	9	0.9 min
100,000	175	342	44	9.35 min
1,000,000	1,441	3,278	443	1 hr 26 min
10,000,000	13,785	31,216	5,017	13 hr 53 min

The original approach would have taken us a few *years* to complete on the 10 million record data set. But the whole computation time for a 10 million by 10 million record run—with encryption, secure comparisons, and matching—takes approximately 14 hours. Now that's a roadrunner!

Final Thoughts

Secure linking solves one of the major challenges in getting access to data from multiple sources. It has a number of common use cases, from de-duplication of databases to linking databases across jurisdictional or organizational boundaries without sharing any personal information. The challenge with such secure protocols is their performance, but with the schemes we've presented here for linking tables, scaling the implementation to larger data sets is feasible on current hardware and doesn't require the use of blocking techniques.

At the end of the secure linking protocol, the only information that's revealed is the identities of the matching records. This is inevitable, and in fact the whole point of the exercise. Therefore, it's important for the Carolers to have the authority or consent to learn the new information they gain from having matched records. Even this requirement can be eliminated by using secure anonymization, whereby the linked data is securely anonymized before it's revealed to the Carolers, but we'll leave that protocol for another book.

References

1. A. Acquisti and R. Gross, "Predicting Social Security Numbers from Public Data," *Proceedings of the National Academy of Science* 106:27 (2009): 10975–10980.

2. P. Paillier, "Public-Key Cryptosystems Based on Composite Degree Residuosity Classes," *Advances in Cryptography—EUROCRYPT '99* (New York: Springer-Verlag, 1999) 223-238.

3. P. Paillier, "Composite-Residuosity Based Cryptography: An Overview," *Cryptobytes* 5:1 (2002): 20–26.

CHAPTER 13

De-Identification and Data Quality: A Clinical Data Warehouse

As is evident from the case studies we've presented, anonymization results in some distortion of the original data. In this chapter we'll discuss the amount of distortion that can be introduced and how it can be effectively managed. We'll focus on de-identification, not masking, because it's de-identification that distorts the variables we might want to use for analysis. The amount of distortion is referred to as "information loss," or conversely "data utility".

Data utility is important for those using anonymized data, because the results of their analyses are critical for informing major care, policy, and investment decisions. Also, the cost of getting access to data is not trivial, making it important to ensure the quality of the data received. We don't want to be wasteful, spending time and money collecting high quality data, to then watch that quality deteriorate through anonymization practices meant to prepare the data for secondary use. What we really want to know is whether the inferences drawn from de-identified data are reliable—that is, are they the same inferences we would draw from the original data?

Useful Data from Useful De-Identification

Although obvious, it's worth repeating that poor de-identification techniques result in less data utility. In fact, that is one key way to evaluate the quality of a de-identification method. Many of the de-identification techniques that we've described are essentially optimization problems. Some optimization methods maximize data utility, while others minimize the risk of re-identification at the expense of data utility. Not all optimization methods are created equal. The goal, of course, is to maximize data utility while meeting the predefined risk thresholds.

The other thing to keep in mind is that errors can occur during the application of de-identification methods. A public example of that was an error in the public use files created by the US Census Bureau that affected inferences about people 65 years and older.[1] In this case, there was a nontrivial reduction in data utility, but only for a segment of the population. When looking at de-identification methods in this chapter, we'll assume that there are no errors and that any loss of utility is a function of the methods used.

Evidence of the impact of de-identification on data utility is mixed. Some studies show little impact,[2] whereas others show a nontrivial impact.[3] There is also evidence that data utility depends on both the de-identification method and the analysis method used.[4,5] Given the mixed reviews, it's more useful to discuss the factors involved in evaluating and interpreting data utility, rather than trying to make overly general statements.

Degrees of Loss

Data utility is not a binary metric: good or bad. Conceptually, there's a spectrum of data utility (remember the Goldilocks principle shown in Figure 2-1 in "Basic Principles" on page 21?). A certain amount of data utility may be acceptable in one instance and not acceptable in another. Let's consider an example of a public data release.

A large health data custodian manages a national registry. This registry has been around for many years, and the internal statisticians have been performing detailed longitudinal analyses on the data for many years. Access to the original data has also been granted to external analysts, after going through a somewhat lengthy screening and approval process. Then, one day, there was a request by the sponsors of the data custodian to create a public version of the registry to allow the large data holdings to be used and made accessible more broadly. The public data would have lower utility than the original registry, given the level of de-identification required. But is that lower utility acceptable?

The users of the public data may be analysts who want to run experiments that internal statisticians would do themselves. The greatest concern these analysts would have is whether they would be able to reproduce the longitudinal analyses done by the internal statisticians, given the lesser utility of a public data release. We can certainly evaluate data utility from that perspective, but there are many other potential data consumers for the public data who might have different requirements.

A public data set can be used in many legitimate ways:

- By app developers as the basis for new tools, and to test them on realistic data
- By students, to learn how to build models
- By computer scientists and statisticians, to do simulations and as examples to illustrate their new algorithms and modeling techniques

- By analysts, to develop protocols and code to include in their proposals for funding to work on the full data set (i.e., to justify going through the lengthy process to get access to the internal data set)
- By the media or other organizations (such as government departments), to produce high-level summaries from the data
- By health care providers, who may want to perform basic benchmarks of their performance
- By data brokers, who want to create aggregate information products for government and industry

For all of these data users, lower data utility may be just fine, because their purposes are different from those of the internal statisticians.

It's important to keep in mind the multitude of users that may want access to a public data set when deciding whether its level of data utility is acceptable. This is of course most pronounced in the case of a public data set, but the issue arises for nonpublic data sets as well.

For public data, to ensure that the needs of all of these stakeholders are addressed, it would be prudent to consult with them during the de-identification process. This can be achieved by creating an advisory body that provides feedback to the de-identification team, and by piloting the anonymization of the data to get real data user feedback.

Workload-Aware De-Identification

Ideally, your de-identification methods are "aware" of the types of analysis that will be performed on the data. If you know that a regression model using age in years is going to be applied, the de-identification should not generalize the age into, say, five-year age intervals. But if the analyst is going to group the age into five-year age bands anyway, because these correspond with known mortality risk bands or something like that, this generalization of age will not have an impact on data utility. Examples of questions you can ask to allow the planned analysis to inform the de-identification are provided in "Questions to Improve Data Utility" on page 189.

Customizing the de-identification parameters to the needs of the analysis is easier to do for nonpublic data, where the data recipient is known. All you need is a conversation or negotiation with the data recipient to match the de-identification methods to the analysis plan, such that variables that are critical for analysis are less likely to be modified (generalized or suppressed) during the de-identification. If the analyst is expected to perform a geospatial analysis, for example, anonymization can ensure that location data is less affected, but subsampling (Chapter 7) could be used to maintain anonymity. In contrast, if the analysis is to detect rare events, subsampling may not be an option during the de-identification, but fuzzing location may be all right. Certain groupings of nominal variables, such as race, ethnicity, language spoken at home, and country of birth, may also be limited if these are critical for the analysis.

If the data recipient is a clinician who doesn't have a data analysis team, limits might be imposed on suppression. Performing imputation (discussed briefly in "Information Loss Metrics" on page 35) to recover information that has been suppressed requires some statistical sophistication, and this might not be something the clinician wants to get into. One of the main advantages of the methodology we've presented in this book is that it allows us to calibrate the de-identification so the data sets are better suited to the needs of the data recipients.

If it's possible to have direct negotiations with the data users, it's definitely worth the time. It will result in higher-quality data for the people that want it. The challenge is often that people are not used to participating in such negotiations and might not be willing to make the effort. Also, many may not understand the issues at hand and the trade-offs involved in different kinds of de-identification. But this relatively minor investment in time can make a big difference in the data utility. It's also a way to manage expectations.

It's not always possible to negotiate directly with a data recipient. A pharmacy that has provided its de-identified data to multiple business partners might not have the capacity to calibrate the data sets to each data user—such workload awareness might not be feasible. But there are a few options to consider:

- You could guess at the types of analyses that are likely to be performed. The planned analyses are often quite simple, consisting of univariate and bivariate statistics and simple cross-tabulations. So the pharmacy could test the results from running these types of analyses before and after de-identification to evaluate data utility. In most cases, the data custodians will have good knowledge of their data and which fields are important for data analysis, which makes them well positioned to make such judgments.
- You could create multiple data sets suited to different analyses. One data set may have more extensive geographic information but less clinical detail, and another data set may have much more clinical information but fewer geographic details.[6] The data setyou provide would depend on the needs of the data user.
- You could ensure high data utility for some common parameters, such as means, standard deviations, correlation and covariance matrices, and basic regression models.[7,8] These parameters are relevant for most analyses that are likely to be performed on the data. The impacts of de-identification on each parameter can be measured using the mean squared error (before and after de-identification).
- You could use general information loss metrics, discussed in "Information Loss Metrics" on page 35. These metrics include the extent of suppression and entropy.

In practice they are relatively good proxies for general distortion to the data, and people can easily understand them.

Of course, you can also use a mix of these options: one type of de-identification for known data users who are willing to negotiate with the data custodian, and a generically de-identified data set for other users.

Questions to Improve Data Utility

You can ask data users a lot of things to better understand the type of analytics that they plan to run on the data. The answers to these questions can help de-identify the data in a manner that will increase its data utility for them. Here are some of these questions, which will help you get the conversation started:

What data do you really need?
: This is probably the most fundamental question to ask. We often see data users asking for all of the variables in a data set, or at least for more variables than they really need or plan to use. Maybe they haven't thought through the analysis methods very carefully yet—they wanted to first see what data they could get. Talking about it with the data users will often result in a nontrivial pruning of the data requested. This is important because fewer variables will mean fewer quasi-identifiers, which leads to higher data utility for the remaining quasi-identifiers after de-identification.

Do you need to perform any geospatial analysis?
: It's important to find out the level of granularity required for any planned geospatial analysis. If a comparative analysis by state is going to be done, state information can be included without any more detailed geospatial data. However, if a hotspot analysis to detect disease outbreaks is to be done, more granular data will be needed. But even if no geospatial analysis is planned, location may be needed for other things —e.g., to link with data about socioeconomic status (SES) from the census (in which case linking the data for the data users, and then dropping the geospatial information in the released data is the easiest option).

Are exact dates needed?
: In many cases exact dates aren't needed. In oncology studies it's often acceptable to convert all dates into intervals from the date of diagnosis (the anchor), and remove the original date of diagnosis itself. Or the analysis can be performed at an annual level to look at year-by-year trends, like changes in the cost of drugs—generalizing dates to year won't affect data utility here. Dates can also be converted to date ranges (e.g., week/year, month/year), depending on what's needed.

Will you be looking for rare events?
: In general, subsampling is a very powerful way to reduce the risk of re-identification for nonpublic data releases. It's a method that you should have in your toolbox. But

if the purpose of the analysis is to detect rare events, or to examine "the long tail," then subsampling would mean losing some of those rare events. By definition, rare events are *rare*, and losing this data is likely to mean losing any chance at statistical significance. In this case, avoid methods that will remove the rare events that are needed.

Can we categorize variables, or group categories into variables?
: To some degree this goes back to the data that is *really* needed, but people often forget about groupings they were planning, or would be willing, to create. They might ask for an education variable (six categories), but actually plan to change the groupings into fewer categories than are present in the original (two categories). The finer distinctions might not be needed to answer questions, or some of the original categories might not have a lot of data in them. These changes can have a big impact on reducing risk, especially for demographics, so it's far better to know this in advance and include it in the de-identification.

Are provider or pharmacy identities necessary?
: Due to the possibility of geoproxy attacks, provider and pharmacy identities increase re-identification risk. It's relatively easy to determine a provider or pharmacy's location from its identity and then predict where the patient lives. For some analyses the provider and pharmacy information is critical, and therefore it's not possible to remove it. But sometimes it is acceptable to remove that information and consequently eliminate the risk of a geoproxy attack.

Can the data recipients perform imputation?
: Performing imputation to recover missing data requires some specialized skills. If the data user or team doesn't have that expertise, then it would be prudent to minimize suppression during de-identification. Otherwise you might be leaving people with data they don't know how to use. If a clinician is planning to do a simple descriptive analysis on the data set and there's no statistician available to help, the impact of missingness might be lost on him. If he's unlikely to perform imputation, or understand the impact of missingness, minimize suppression.

Would you be willing to impose additional controls?
: One way to increase data utility is to increase the risk threshold so that less de-identification is required. You can do this by improving the mitigating controls, if there's a willingness to put in place stronger security and privacy practices. If there's time, it's helpful to show data users what data they would get with the current versus the improved mitigating controls. That way they can decide whether it's worth the effort for them to strengthen their security and privacy practices.

Is it possible to strengthen the data sharing agreement?
: This is another way to increase the risk threshold so that less de-identification is required. The first measure we would suggest, and the first that we look for, is that the data sharing agreement has a provision in place that prohibits re-identification,

to reduce motives and capacity. This would increase the risk threshold so that less de-identification is required.

A Clinical Data Warehouse

We created an anonymized data warehouse for analytics purposes from an EMR database, which we'll use to illustrate ways to evaluate data quality. A wide range of analyses may be performed on the data, including post-marketing surveillance of drugs, public health surveillance, and determining the number of patients who meet screening criteria for clinical trials. Therefore, the anonymized data had to meet a broad range of needs.

The EMR database covered 535,595 patients in Ontario, with 5,850 providers working in 2,664 clinics across the province. The data itself included all clinical encounters, billing information, claims (which included diagnosis and procedures), drugs prescribed, laboratory data that was sent to the EMR database for all tests ordered by the providers, and basic demographics on the patients. A total of 75 tables from the EMR database were anonymized. The remaining tables (more than 200 of them) were log tables or contained look-up and reference information that didn't have personally identifiying information.

The data custodian was the EMR vendor and the data recipient was providing analytics services. As part of the anonymization process, we answered the set of questions in "Questions to Improve Data Utility" on page 189 to maximize data quality. The responses to these questions, in Table 13-1, suggest that subsampling would not be a good approach to use, and that retaining date fidelity is important.

Table 13-1. Q&A on the data quality for the anonymization of the EMR database.

The Q	And the A
What data do you *really* need?	For the purpose of analytics, all of the data in the EMR database is needed because data requests are expected to vary quite a bit.
Do you need to perform any geospatial analysis?	Some geospatial analysis is anticipated, so patient location information is important.
Are *exact* dates needed?	Yes, many of the anticipated analyses will be date-based (such as how many prescriptions were written for a discontinued drug, where a key date would be the date the drug was discontinued).
Will you be looking for rare events?	The analysis of rare events is very likely because, for example, adverse events from drugs are expected to be quite rare.
Can we categorize variables, or group categories into variables?	It's difficult to anticipate in advance all of the possible analyses and therefore which categories will be most relevant.
Are provider or pharmacy identities necessary?	These identities are not necessary.
Do the data recipients have the ability to perform imputation?	Yes, the data recipient has sophisticated statistical analysis capabilities.

The Q	And the A
Would you be willing to impose additional controls?	Yes, and significant controls have been put in place already.
Is it possible to strengthen the data sharing agreement?	Yes, but a very strong data sharing agreement is already in place.

To evaluate data quality after anonymization, we first looked at two study protocols. The protocols described real surveillance analyses that the data recipient was looking to perform, and were chosen to produce small counts because they would be the ones most likely affected by anonymization. Therefore, such data quality tests provide a stringent and realistic evaluation of the impact of anonymization. What the data recipient wanted to know was whether the computed statistics on the data before and after anonymization were the same, to ensure they would get the same basic results after anonymization.

After looking at two study protocols, we then evaluated the impact of date shifting on the distribution of events in the EMR database. Given the importance of dates for the anticipated analyses that will be performed on the data warehouse, a detailed understanding of the impact of date shifting is necessary.

GI Protocol

The first study protocol considered patients that had at least one gastrointestinal (GI) event after taking nonsteroidal anti-inflammatory drugs (NSAID's) for the first time, with or without proton pump inhibitor (PPI) drugs. Drugs prescribed by the physician are automatically recorded in the EMR database. The following define the patient inclusion criteria:

- Had taken one of the NSAIDs for the first time in 2011 (i.e., no prescriptions for one of these in 2010).
- Has never taken one of the PPIs prior to first NSAID.
- Has a diagnosis of any of the following ICD-9 codes in 2011: 714 (rheumatoid arthritis), 715 (osteoarthritis), 720 (ankylosing spondylitis), 729 (such as myalgia and myositis), 739 (nonallopathic lesions), and 781 (symptoms involving nervous and musculoskeletal systems).

Two arms were defined, and the purpose of the analysis was to compare the number of patients in each arm:

Arm 1

A patient who had NSAID initiated and did *not* get a PPI prescribed at the same visit as the NSAID initiated.

Arm 2

A patient who had an NSAID initiated and *did* get a PPI prescribed at the same visit as the NSAID initiated.

The measured outcomes from the EMR database were defined as:

- Arm 1 outcome: Number of GI events from NSAID initiation to April 2013.
- Arm 2 outcome: Number of GI events from NSAID initiation plus PPI to April 2013.

A GI event is any of the following ICD-9 codes: 530 (diseases of esophagus), 531 (gastric ulcer), 534 (gastrojejunal ulcer), 535 (acute gastritis), 536 (disorders of function of stomach), 537 (disorders of stomach and duodenum), and 553 (gastritis and duodenitis).

This protocol has a limitation in that the EMR database captures the prescription, but that does not necessarily mean that the patient has taken the drug. The patient may not have gone to a pharmacy to order the drug, and this can't be determined without information on dispensation (which is not avaible from the EMR database). Information on how well the patient complied with the instructions for taking their prescription drugs was also not available.

The results comparing the two arms in Table 13-2 show that anonymization had little impact on the raw counts of GI events. Only the first arm of the protocol was affected at all, and not much at that, whereas the second arm produced exactly the same results. The substantive conclusions are not affected by anonymization.

Table 13-2. GI counts before and after anonymization.

ARM	GI Before	GI After
1	73	78
2	8	8

Chlamydia Protocol

The purpose of the second study protocol was to determine the chlamydia screening and positivity rates for sexually active females from 14 to 24 years of age, inclusive. The Canadian government has recently published screening guidelines for chlamydia requiring that all sexually active young females be screened for the disease.[9]

There are three reasons why patients may be tested for chlamydia:

- The patient presents with symptoms.
- The patient requests testing because of an exposure or a concern.

- The physician offers testing for screening purposes in an asymptomatic person.

By definition, patients tested under (1) and (2) are sexually active, and would be eligible for screening if they're under 25 years of age. Under condition (3), a patient would be tested only if the physician is following recommended screening practices (assuming the patient is sexually active).

The EMR database from which the data was extracted received laboratory results automatically for tests ordered by the physician. The largest laboratories that conduct chlamydia testing in the covered geographies provided this data, so we expected the measurements to provide good coverage of chlamydia testing for this population.

Two caveats are worth mentioning:

- The estimates do not include testing performed by public health clinics and anonymous testing.
- The estimates are based on all females rather than those who are sexually active. The latter number is difficult to determine because younger females may be less willing to divulge this information, even with their own doctor, and using birth control prescriptions would provide an incomplete picture.

These considerations probably deflate the estimates, because the denominator we used is higher than it would be if the estimates could account for those lapses.

We calculated the opportunisitic screening (or testing) rate and the positivity rate detected from visits for one year periods from 2007/06/01 to 2013/06/01, for female patients aged 14-24 inclusive. Opportunistic screening means the person is screened when the opportunity arises, which in this case is a visit to a doctor's office.

A female with a birth date in the appropriate study year was counted once in her age group if she visited the doctor at least once that year. So if she was born in 1997/01/01 (happy New Year!), then she would be counted as 14 in the study year 2010/06/01 to 2011/06/01 (study year 2011 for short). We didn't want to double dip by counting a person that had a doctor's visit before and after her birthdate, since the guidelines say they need to be screened only once during the study period. But that New Year's girl would also be counted as 15 in study year 2012, and 16 in study year 2013. Now if she was screened multiple times in a study year then she was only counted once for that year (again, no double dipping).

The overall results in Table 13-3 show no meaningful differences before and after anonymization. None of the rates were found to be different by a statistically significant amount (differences were evaluated as two independent samples, given that patient age was randomized). There are no noticeable trends in screening over time. For whatever reason, the screening rate in 2010 was at a significant low, which resulted in a small population from which to measure the positivity rate that year. So although the positiviy rate seems very different, the error in this estimate is much higher.

Table 13-3. Overall chlamydia rates before and after anonymization over six years.

Year	Age Group	Screening Before	Screening After	Positivity Before	Positivity After
2008	14-24	1,080/10,607 (10%)	1,135/10,638 (11%)	77/1,080 (7.1%)	78/1,135 (6.9%)
2009	14-24	1,056/11,442 (9.2%)	1,084/11,358 (9.5%)	185/1,056 (18%)	186/1,084 (17%)
2010	14-24	229/13,043 (1.8%)	243/13,110 (1.9%)	67/229 (29%)	75/243 (31%)
2011	14-24	1,059/13,414 (7.9%)	1,103/13,558 (8.1%)	135/1,059 (13%)	132/1,103 (12%)
2012	14-24	1,226/13,672 (9.0%)	1,305/13,637 (9.6%)	97/1,226 (7.9%)	107/1,305 (8.2%)
2013	14-24	683/14,308 (4.8%)	681/14,214 (4.8%)	66/683 (9.7%)	69/681 (10%)

We further split the results up by two-year age groups to see how they would fare, but that made for too many tables to show here. Instead, we summarize the rates in Figure 13-1 and Figure 13-2 (the vertical bars are 95% confidence intervals). This also gives us the chance to see if there's an interesting trend over time (although in truth, the Mann-Kendall test failed to reject the null hypothesis of no trend, so we have no statistical evidence that suggests a trend).

To dig a little deeper, let's take a look at the specific results for the last year in Table 13-4. Only one rate was found to be different by a statistically significant amount, indicated by a * in the table (differences were evaluated as two independent samples, given that patient age was randomized). This means that the differences otherwise shown in the results are those that are expected from random variation. As populations get smaller, variability increases, which is why the pooled results in Table 13-3 seem better.

Table 13-4. Chlamydia rates by 2-year age groups before and after anonymization

Year	Age Group	Screening Before	Screening After	Positivity Before	Positivity After
2013	14-15	8/1,130 (0.7%)	16/1,391 (1.1%)	1/8 (13%)	5/16 (31%)
2013	16-17	24/1,587 (1.5%)	14/1,349 (1.0%)	4/24 (17%)	1/14 (7.1%)
2013	18-19	81/2,228 (3.6%)	137/2,767 (5.0%)*	7/81 (8.6%)	11/137 (8.0%)
2013	20-21	189/3,113 (6.1%)	158/3,043 (5.2%)	17/189 (9.0%)	22/158 (14%)
2013	22-23	236/3,996 (5.9%)	205/3,426 (6.0%)	26/236 (11%)	19/205 (9.3%)
2013	24	143/2,198 (6.5%)	149/2,198 (6.8%)	10/142 (7.0%)	11/149 (7.4%)

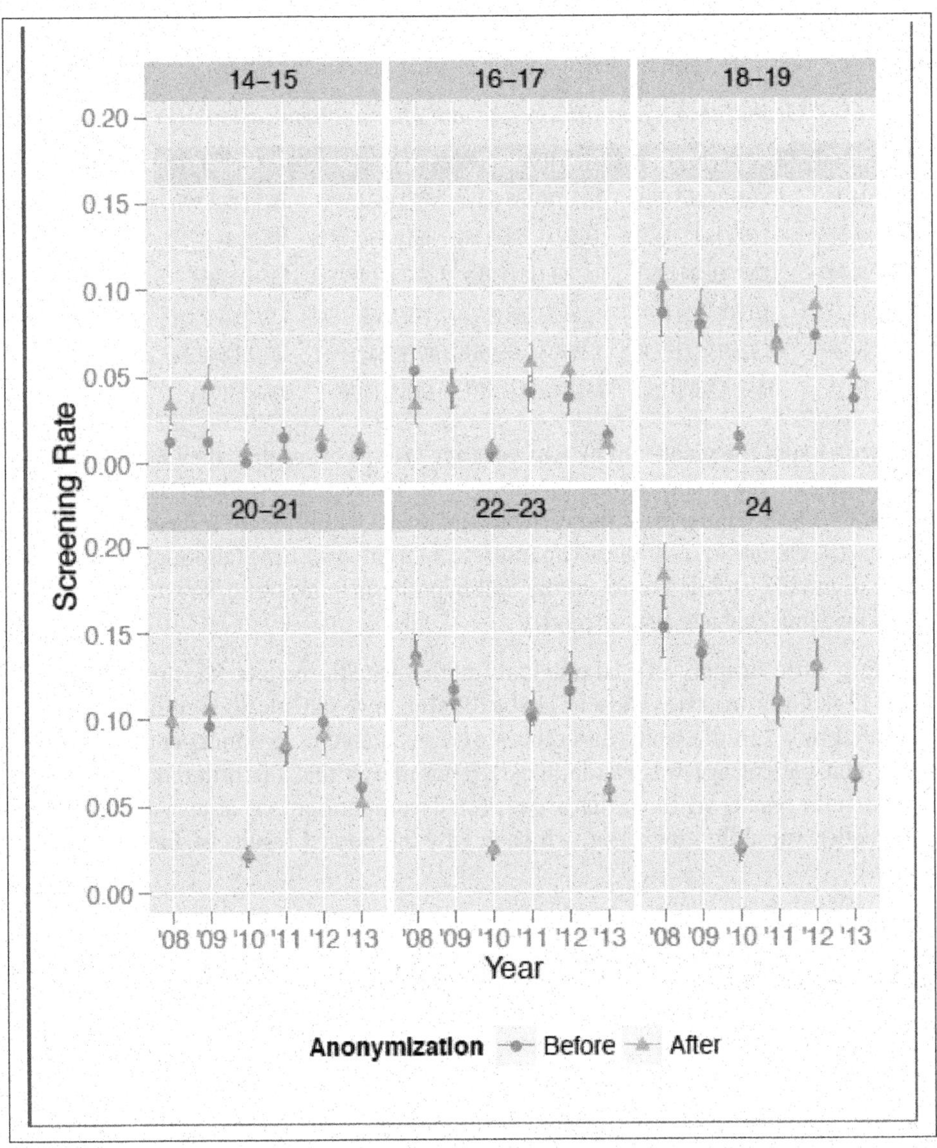

Figure 13-1. Chlamydia screening rates by 2-year age groups before and after anonymization. Not very trendy.

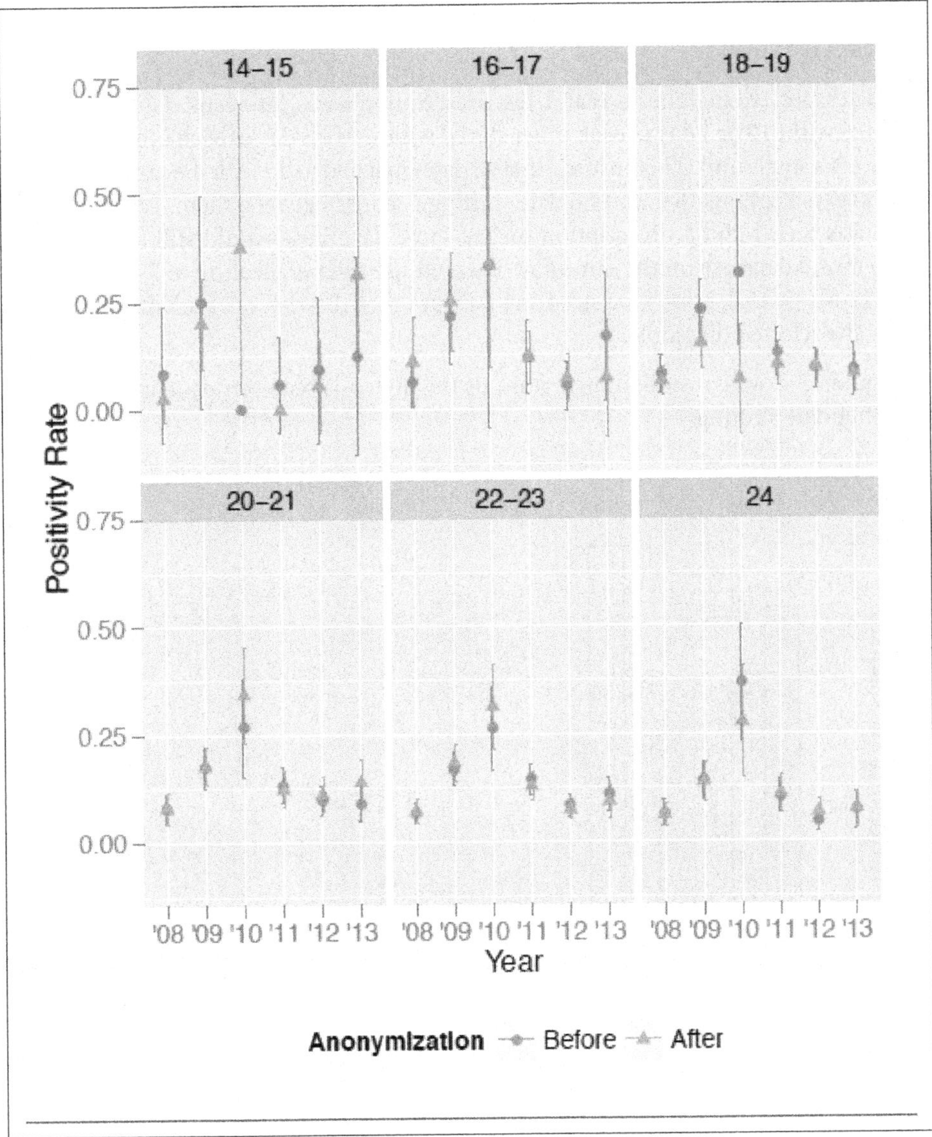

Figure 13-2. Chlamydia positivity rates by 2-year age groups before and after anonymization. Up, down, all around!

Date Shifting

Date shifting was performed on all dates in the EMR database. By its very construction, the order of events is preserved by date shifting. But the distribution across all dates may change—order by patient is preservered, not the order between patients. How does this affect data quality?

The dates affected include all visit dates, prescription dates, lab result dates, and so on. All dates within 0 or 1 day of each other stayed within 0 or 1 day of each other, as though they were a single unit. This ensured that all dates that had to do with the same encounter were always kept together and no date shifting occured between them. For example, if there was a visit and a prescription on the same day, these would still appear in the anonymized database on the same day. Then we use a generalization of 7-day intervals (e.g., [2-8], [9-15]), which we needed to ensure that the risk of re-identification was below the selected threshold.

In Figure 13-3 we consider a histogram of the intervals between patient dates before and after date shifting.

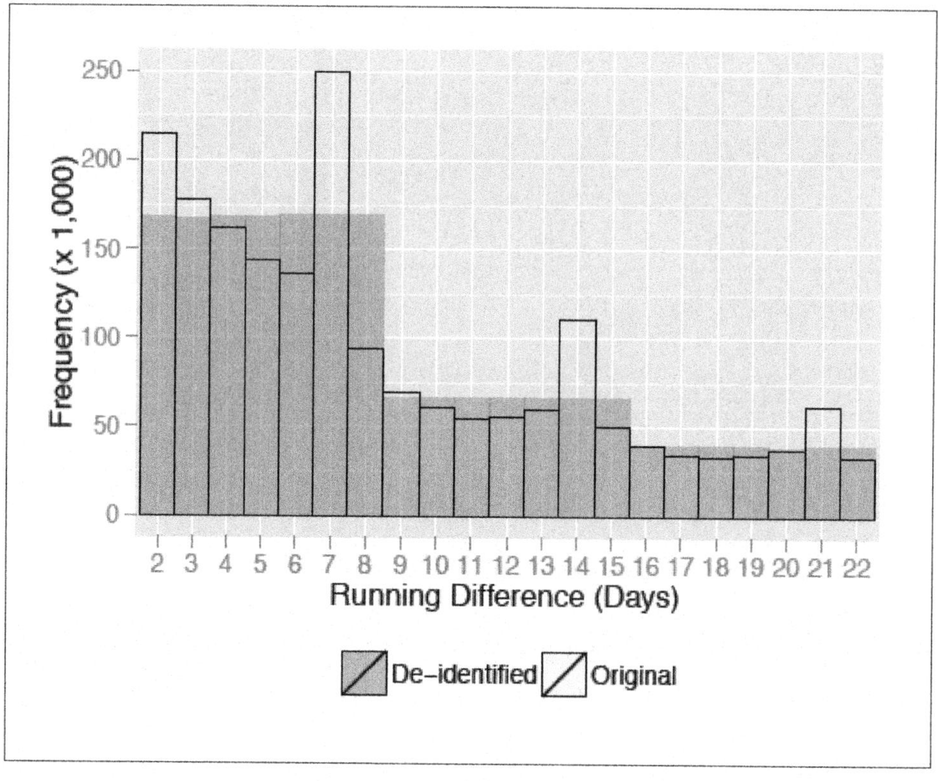

Figure 13-3. Histogram of the running difference between dates before and after date shifting, for any and all dates that didn't occur on the same or next day

This is for dates consolidated into a single column for the sake of multi-table date shifting. We use a "running difference" between dates, so that two rows with the same date, for the same patient, will have a difference of 0 days. That way we don't count the same date twice. The frequency of 0 and 1 day don't change, because they have not been randomized, so we drop their counts from the histogram for the sake of clarity.

From [2-8], the running difference after date shifting has been averaged out across all days. Similarly from [9-15]. The reason for this averaging is that we sample the generalized intervals from a uniform distribution on [2-8], and similarly [9-15]. By randomly sampling within the generalized interval, an adversary has no way to know the actual interval between events for that patient.

We also see this from the frequency table of exact counts in Table 13-5. That is, the frequency after date shifting is the mean frequency over the respective generalized interval. For example, for the generalized interval [2-8], we sum the frequency for intervals 2 to 8 and get a mean frequency of 168,860, which very closely matches the frequency after date shifting of any one interval of 2 up to 8. Similarly for the generalized interval [9-15]. Also note that the average change across all of the intervals is zero.

Table 13-5. Frequency of the running difference before and after date shifting.

Difference (Days)	Generalized	Frequency Before	Frequency After
0	0	13,054,537	13,054,537
1	1	320,532	320,532
2	[2-8]	215,552	168,746
3	[2-8]	178,135	167,990
4	[2-8]	162,209	168,821
5	[2-8]	144,472	168,714
6	[2-8]	136,564	169,083
7	[2-8]	250,579	169,733
8	[2-8]	94,510	169,034
9	[9-15]	70,830	66,386
10	[9-15]	61,129	66,826
11	[9-15]	55,405	66,786
12	[9-15]	56,772	66,714
13	[9-15]	60,856	66,738
14	[9-15]	111,978	66,747
15	[9-15]	50,489	66,262

Next, in Figure 13-4, we consider a histogram of patient length of service (LOS), which we define as the sum of a patient's running difference. This means that the LOS for a patient is the total period that the patient has had dates recorded in their EHR—it's the interval from their first recorded healthcare service to their very last (from encounters, lab tests, even the date of prescriptions refills).

As we can see from the first hundred days, the number of patients with specific LOS is very similar to the original data. The "spikes" at multiples of 7 days in the original data are the same we saw in the previous histogram, and are lost in the de-identified data due to the averaging caused by uniform sampling. We used a Kolmogorov-Smirnov test for shape comparison and found no statistically significant difference between the histograms.[10]

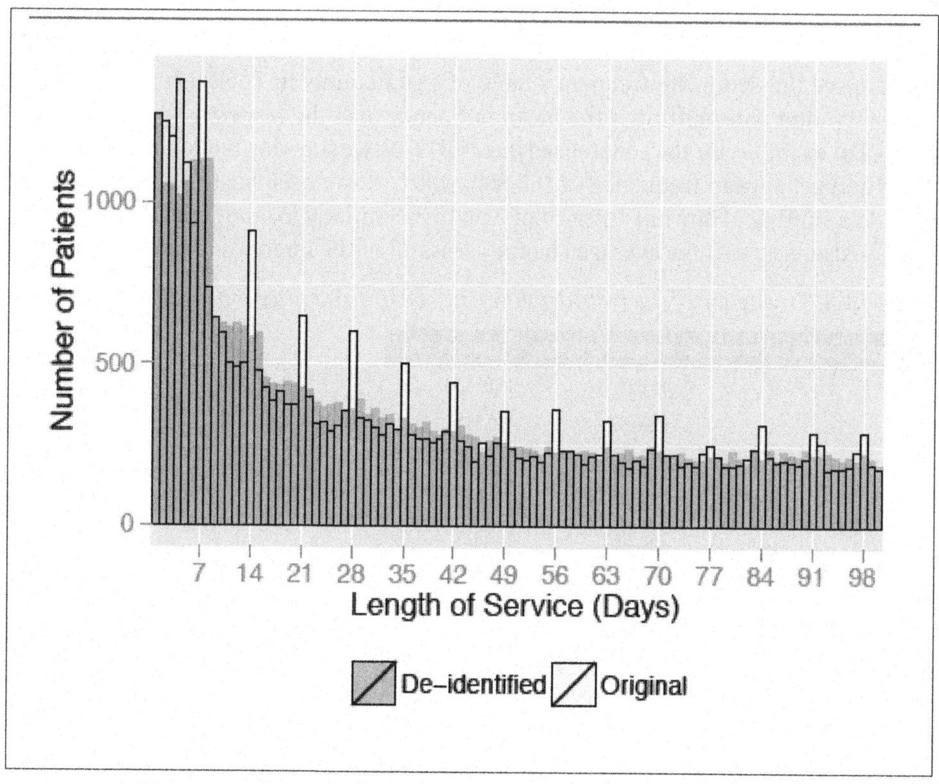

Figure 13-4. Histogram of LOS before and after date shifting

Although not shown, the tail of the histogram for LOS over 100 days looks the same as what we see in this histogram from about 50 to 100 days (i.e., a long tail that's pretty flat, before and after anonymization). Because the whole LOS is affected, since it's the sum of the running difference, does that mean that some patients will now have events in the future? If we consider a cut-off of July 15th, 2013 as the definition of "today," less than 0.03% of the 24 million dates were shifted into the future. Of course, we're not counting dates that were already in the future.

We can also look at the difference in LOS before and after de-identification to see whether date shifting lengthens or shortens the LOS for patients. Remember that we've defined LOS as the sum of the running difference between a patient's sequence of dates. So if a patient has LOS of 100 days before date shifting, and LOS of 90 days after date shifting (because we've de-identified the running difference), the difference in LOS is -10 days (i.e., LOS was shortened by 10 days).

This is something we want to quantify across all patients so that we can evaluate the variation in LOS before and after date shifting. There's no point including patients with only one date (i.e., a running difference of only 0, and LOS of 0), because no date shifting would have been applied to their sequence of dates, so we removed them from consideration.

We expect the mean shift in dates to be zero, meaning LOS will be the same before and after date shifting. What we find, in Figure 13-5, is exactly that: the mean difference in LOS before and after date shifting is 0.2 days.

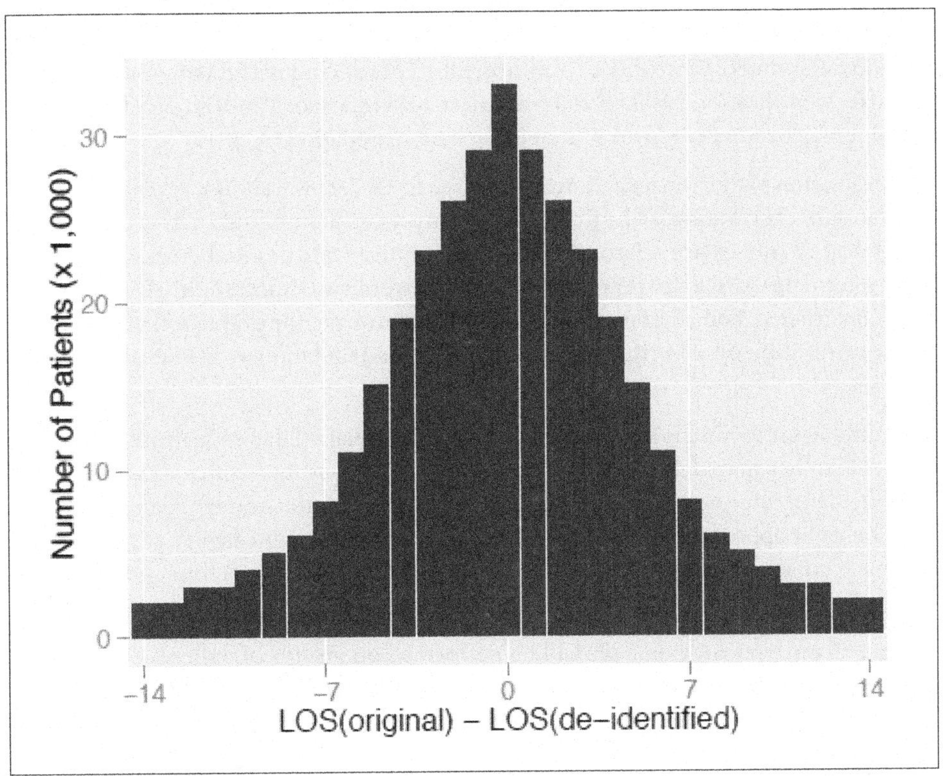

Figure 13-5. Histogram of the difference in length of service before and after date shifting (for 90% of patients)

Not only that, but 80% of patients have an LOS after date shifting that is within plus or minus 9 days of the original LOS, 90% within plus or minus 14 days, and 95% within plus or minus 20 days of the original LOS (due to long tails in the distribution). Also remember that this analysis considered all dates across the full period covered by the database.

The difference in LOS follows a normal distribution for the 90% of patients shown in the histogram. This is a good thing because it shows that the difference in LOS is randomly generated in a natural way that we can understand. The tails of the distribution are long, but this is also something we commonly see in real data, and that we expected (due to biases in the sequence of dates for these patients). It seems fair to say that date shifting has retained the overall characteristics and truthfulness of dates.

Final Thoughts

The amount of change made by de-identification to data utility is important, and very context-driven. All stakeholders need to provide input on what is most important to them, be it data utility or privacy. It's not easy to balance the needs of everyone involved, but good communication and a commitment to producing useful data that keeps the risk of re-identification low is all you really need to get started. It's not an easy negotiation —and it may be iterative—but it is an important negotiation to have.

Our evaluation of the impact on a real and large EMR data warehouse reveals a number of important observations. The first is that, in practice, many of the analyses performed on clinical databases are relatively simple descriptive statistics and cross-tabulations. Only when data is disclosed for research purposes would we expect sophisticated models to be constructed. For general-purpose databases, however, the evaluation of the impact of anonymization on descritpive statistics and cross-tabulations will likely cover most analyses.

A second factor to note is that when evaluating data quality, the evaluations need to be statistical rather than deterministic. Traditional quality assurance on a database would test whether a value before anonymization is the same as after anonymization. But this isn't the right approach for anonymized data—the values will often change. A better approach compares the relevant statisical properties of the data before and after anonymization.

Almost all analyses on a data set will be performed on groups of patients. This means that looking at how anonymizatiom affects a single patient will not be informative. Evaluations of data quality must therefore consider groups of patients and the relevant statistics computed on them.

References

1. J. Alexander, M. Davern, and B. Stevenson, "Inaccurate Age and Sex Data in the Census PUMS Files: Evidence and Implications," NBER Working Paper No. 15703 (Cambridge, MA: National Bureau of Economic Research, 2010).

2. A. Kennickell and J. Lane, "Measuring the Impact of Data Protection Techniques on Data Utility: Evidence from the Survey of Consumer Finances," in *Privacy in Statistical Databases*, ed. J. Domingo-Ferrer and L. Franconi (Berlin: Springer, 2006), 291–303.

3. K. Purdam and M. Elliot, "A Case Study of the Impact of Statistical Disclosure Control on Data Quality in the Individual UK Samples of Anonymised Records," *Environment and Planning A* 39:5 (2007): 1101–1118.

4. S. Lechner and W. Pohlmeier, "To Blank or Not to Blank? A Comparison of the Effects of Disclosure Limitation Methods on Nonlinear Regression Estimates," in *Privacy in Statistical Databases*, ed. J. Domingo-Ferrer and V. Torra (Berlin: Springer, 2004), 187–200.

5. L. H. Cox and J. J. Kim, "Effects of Rounding on the Quality and Confidentiality of Statistical Data," in *Privacy in Statistical Databases*, ed. J. Domingo-Ferrer and L. Franconi (Berlin: Springer, 2006), 48–56.

6. K. El Emam, D. Paton, F. Dankar, and G. Koru, "De-identifying a Public Use Microdata File from the Canadian National Discharge Abstract Database," *BMC Medical Informatics and Decision Making* 11:53 (2011).

7. W. E. Winkler, "Methods and Analyses for Determining Quality," in *Proceedings of the 2nd International Workshop on Information Quality in Information Systems* (Baltimore, MD: ACM, 2005), 3

8. Josep Domingo-Ferrer and Vicenç Torra, "Disclosure Control Methods and Information Loss for Microdata," in *Confidentiality Disclosure and Data Access: Theory and Practical Applications for Statistical Agencies*, ed. P. Doyle, J. Lane, J. Theeuwes, and L. Zayatz (Amsterdam: Elsevier Science, 2001), 91–110.

9. Public Health Agency of Canada. Canadian Guidelines on Sexually Transmitted Infections. 2008.

10. F. Porter, "Testing Consistency of Two Histograms," *arXiv* (2008):0804.0380.

Index

A

B

We'd like to hear your suggestions for improving our indexes. Send email to index@oreilly.com.

C

D

E

F

G

H

I

J

K

L

M

N

O

P

Q

R

S

T

U

V

W

Z

About the Authors

Dr. Khaled El Emam is an Associate Professor at the University of Ottawa, Faculty of Medicine, a senior investigator at the Children's Hospital of Eastern Ontario Research Institute, and a Canada Research Chair in Electronic Health Information at the University of Ottawa. He is also the Founder and CEO of Privacy Analytics, Inc. His main area of research is developing techniques for health data de-identification/anonymization and secure computation protocols for health research and public health purposes. He has made many contributions to the health privacy area.

Luk Arbuckle has been crunching numbers for a decade. He originally plied his trade in the area of image processing and analysis, and then in the area of applied statistics. Since joining the Electronic Health Information Laboratory (EHIL) at the CHEO Research Institute he has worked on methods to de-identify health data, participated in the development and evaluation of secure computation protocols, and provided all manner of statistical support. As a consultant with Privacy Analytics, he has also been heavily involved in conducting risk analyses on the re-identification of patients in health data.

Colophon

The animals on the cover of *Anonymizing Health Data* are Atlantic Herring (*Clupea harengus*), one of the most abundant fish species in the entire world. They can be found on both sides of the Atlantic Ocean and congregate in schools that can include hundreds of thousands of individuals.

These silver fish grow quickly and can reach 14 inches in length. They can live up to 15 years and females lay as many as 200,000 eggs over their lives. Herring play a key role in the food web of the northwest Atlantic Ocean: bottom-dwelling fish like flounder, cod, and haddock feed on herring eggs, and juvenile herring are preyed upon by dolphins, sharks, skates, sea lions, squid, orca whales, and sea birds.

Despite being so important to the ecology of the ocean, the herring population has suffered from overfishing in the past. The lowest point for the Atlantic herring came during the 1960s when foreign fleets began harvesting herring and decimated the population within ten years. In 1976, Congress passed the Magnuson-Stevens Act to regulate domestic fisheries, and the Atlantic herring population has made a great resurgence since then.

Herring fisheries are especially important in the American northeast, where the fish are sold frozen, salted, canned as sardines, or in bulk as bait for lobster and tuna fishermen. In 2011, the total herring harvest was worth over $24 million. Fisheries in New England and Canada do especially well because herring tend to congregate near the coast in the cold waters of the Gulf of Maine and Gulf of St. Lawrence. As long as the current regulations on fisheries stand, the Atlantic herring will continue to be a very important member of both the Atlantic Ocean's ecosystem and our worldwide economy.

The cover image is from Brockhaus's *Lexikon*. The cover fonts are URW Typewriter and Guardian Sans. The text font is Adobe Minion Pro; the heading font is Adobe Myriad Condensed; and the code font is Dalton Maag's Ubuntu Mono.

CPSIA information can be obtained
at www.ICGtesting.com
Printed in the USA
BVOW09s1255081116
467251BV00007B/40/P